# The
# Whole Life
# Fertility
# Plan

# The Whole Life Fertility Plan

Understanding What Affects
Your Fertility To Help You Get Pregnant
When You Want To

Kyra Phillips
+
Jamie Grifo, MD, PhD

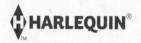

The Whole Life Fertility Plan: Understanding What Affects Your Fertility To Help You Get Pregnant When You Want To

ISBN-13: 978-0-373-89296-9

The health advice presented in this book is intended only as an informative resource guide to help you make informed decisions; it is not meant to replace the advice of a physician or to serve as a guide to self-treatment. Always seek competent medical help for any health condition or if there is any question about the appropriateness of a procedure or health recommendation.

Phillips, Kyra.
  The whole life fertility plan : understanding what affects your fertility to help you get pregnant when you want to / by Kyra Phillips and Dr. Jamie Grifo, MD, PhD.
     pages cm
  Includes bibliographical references and index.
  ISBN 978-0-373-89296-9 (hardback)
1. Conception—Popular works. 2. Fertility, Human—Popular works. 3. Infertility—Alternative treatment—Popular works.  I. Grifo, Jamie. II. Title.
  RG133.P45 2015
  618.1'78—dc23
                2014034980

www.Harlequin.com

**Printed in U.S.A.**

## From Kyra...

I dedicate this book to my husband, JD. Not only did you provide me with the super sperm that makes our twins brilliant, it was you who encouraged and inspired me and Jamie to write this book. Thank you for the gift of motherhood, family and the deepest love I have ever known.

## From Jamie...

I dedicate this book to my family:

My wife Anne, who encouraged me to write a book I would never have been able to without her support and encouragement.

My five amazing children: Jamie, Chris, Maggie, Isabella and Biagia, whom I dearly love and who challenge me, teach me, humble me and terrify me.

My family of six sisters, one brother, my parents and the village of others who raised us.

Last but not least to my patients, who allow me the privilege of helping them build their families so I can make a small difference in this very big world—one loved, cherished and appreciated baby at a time.

# Contents

# Preface:
## Our Stories

## Kyra's Story

The turning point in my life was the day my house flooded.

I was away on assignment, which was where I usually was at the time. I was born to be a reporter, and by that I mean I started up an unauthorized school newspaper in the fourth grade. My best friend in class had a father who was a piano tuner, and she once told me that he tuned Dr. Seuss's piano, so I convinced her that it would be a very good idea if the two of us sneaked into his office to find Dr. Seuss's phone number so I could interview him for my newspaper.

"Where did you get this number?"

I was unprepared for the tenor of hostility I detected on the other end from one Theodore Geisel.

"Sir, I got it from my friend's dad and I wanted to know if I could interview you for the very first issue of Valencia Park Elementary School's newspaper, which I have founded myself."

I expected him to congratulate me on my moxie and possibly suggest that I come over for lunch and shadow him for a day as he wrote his next book.

"What an intrepid little reporter you are!" he would say. "You have a bright future ahead of you."

Instead he said, "You have five minutes." Now, if I could find any record whatsoever of that interview, I might not be able to make this assertion, but since there is no proof otherwise, I'm declaring that it was the most poignant five-minute interview of his life. From that point on, I was hooked.

## Career Woman

I worked my way up from intrepid elementary school newspaper reporter to CNN, which was when I truly felt that I had arrived. My career was going wonderfully, but it became suddenly clear to me at age thirty that my girlfriends were getting married and I wasn't. I wanted to be the woman who had it all, and having it all meant a husband and kids in addition to the great career. Although I wasn't ready for changing diapers just yet, I did think it was time to get on the path. So I got married.

I mean, it wasn't entirely impulsive—I didn't just grab some random guy who happened to be walking by the nearest Vegas courthouse—but it probably wasn't the wisest decision of my life. Even so, for the first few years, it was good. He wanted to have a family right away but I didn't, so we sort of compromised: We didn't try, but we didn't use birth control, either. I hoped Mother Nature would recognize that this was not the right timing and go bless some other young woman's womb and leave mine alone for a while. I was too interested in traveling and reporting at the time.

I spent a month in Antarctica in 2002 working on a documentary about the science and danger on Earth's most frigid continent, tracing the steps of the famous explorer Sir Ernest Shackleton. I built and slept in an igloo, rappelled down glaciers, introduced viewers to rare penguin colonies and got to report on some of the continent's most fascinating scientific discoveries.

You know what I wasn't thinking about? Babies. I was even kind of judgy about the women my age who were having babies. Girlfriends who used to be up for drinking and dancing all night long now said, "Oh, but little Joey will be so out of sorts if I'm not here when he goes to bed" or "I have to be up early to take Maya to the zoo tomorrow." I was thinking, *These poor women. Those kids have taken over their whole identities. They don't even remember how to have fun anymore.*

I also did not understand how certain women in my office could bail out of work early because of something-or-other with their kids. *Don't you get it?* I thought. *You have a great job! How could you blow it by not being committed to it?*

I'm telling you, I was a jerk. Not to anyone's face, but in my own brain I was. There was plenty of time to be saddled with little children later, I figured. I wanted to suck out all the marrow of life, as Henry David Thoreau put it, and I sure couldn't do that with a diaper bag slung over my shoulder.

My family was great about staying out of my ovaries and encouraging me to follow whatever path I chose—in fact, they seemed to admire my independence and hadn't bugged me about getting married, either—but this one coworker seemed to be on a personal mission to make me reproduce as soon as possible.

"Kyra, you would be a great mom. You need to hurry up and have a baby. You really can have it all. I don't know what you're waiting for."

"Yeah, uh-huh," I said sagely.

"I'm making it work. I have it all," she said. "You can, too!"

*Yeah, sure. But are you getting sent on this great interview on the other side of the world? Are you covering the exciting assignments? No. That would be me, because you have to be back in time to lead the Daisy troop. Sucker.*

This conversation occurred nearly every time she caught me sitting in the makeup chair. I couldn't get up and walk away, so it was the perfect time to grill me. I just replied "Yeah, uh-huh" and gave noncommittal answers while I mentally rolled my eyes.

When the war in Iraq began, I reported as an embedded journalist aboard the *USS Abraham Lincoln* and from the ground once the U.S. military moved in. I learned about the strong faith of the Iraqi people, and about how to survive on nothing. Even our own military had very meager accommodations and supplies. You had to find a way to live without nearly any of the comforts of home—the things you'd always taken for granted. It was in this place of lack and nothingness that my spirit took a giant leap forward. I slept well. I got back to basics and I talked to people. It felt like important work, and I received many awards for it.

I felt good about myself as a person and as a woman. I wasn't having anxious chats with my uterus about when we were going to get it together. Maybe I *should* have been, but I didn't know that. I figured I was in good shape, still looked young and had plenty of time. But then my marriage fell apart, which you probably saw coming, because "I'm thirty and I think I'm falling behind schedule" is a terrible reason to get married and there was finally no denying that anymore.

Things got really, really, really bad in a short period of time. Ugly bad. We got a divorce in 2007, which left me feeling not only brokenhearted, but as though I was "off the path." Now I was even more behind schedule because I had to start over.

A friend of mine with the same "starting over" fear stayed in an abusive marriage just because she wanted to have three kids and she was afraid it would take too long to find someone new and get settled before it was too late. She felt as if she needed to start having kids soon if she was going to have enough time to have all three, and that became temporarily more important to her than whether or not the guy would actually be a good husband or parent.

She snapped out of it after he abused her in front of their first (and what would be their only) baby. I wonder, though, if she had known more about her options, would she have left him sooner?

We women are under enough pressure as it is. We're still expected to be the more domestic ones in a couple, while also balancing work and other responsibilities. We're expected to walk the fine line between being powerful and being traditionally feminine. And then we put this unnecessary pressure onto ourselves by expecting our life to run according to a perfect schedule. In my friend's case, her life was supposed to go like this: marriage at twenty-seven, first baby at twenty-eight, second at thirty-one, third at thirty-four. Three years apart, each one, and still young enough to feel that she'd have plenty of energy to keep up with them.

Unfortunately, our lives often don't follow our schedules. No one schedules fertility problems into the mix, and how can you plan for marital troubles, or when you'll meet the right guy, or when you'll get laid off from your job—or promoted? Or when a loved one will get ill and need you? Ignoring our conscience and forging ahead with our plans usually gets us in trouble. You have to be adaptable, especially when it comes to building a family.

But an important lesson I hope to teach you is this: Don't let anyone—including yourself—pressure you into having a baby. If you don't think this is the right time, or the right partner, or the right situation, then wait. Follow what we're going to teach you about preserving your fertility and the options that are available to you, and then wait until it does feel right. It's important for you to feel happy and secure about your decision, which should also help your future child feel safe and loved.

I can tell you now that if I had pressured myself into having kids sooner, it would have been the wrong decision. Not only would I have been with the wrong guy, but I also would have resented the fact that I hadn't yet done all the things I wanted to do as a single person, before someone else became dependent on me. There is something to be said for "sowing your wild oats." And my oats were pretty wild. They weren't your average oatmeal-type oats, no siree. They were the oats that escaped from the grocery shelves and went out partying with the spicy nachos.

So if people are bugging you about having kids, smile and nod or tell them to back off—whatever's more your style.

## The Flood

Sometimes, with major life events, you "just know." People say you'll "just know" when you meet the person you're supposed to spend your life with. I didn't. Oops. But I did know when I was ready to have a baby.

I returned from three months in Baghdad and then CNN sent me straight to New York to fill in for a morning anchor who was out on maternity leave. It was a great move to keep me occupied and away from the home that would remind me of my ex. I did not particularly like my coanchor, a distant and egotistical man named John Roberts, but whatever.

He never let me announce my own name at the opening of the show. It was always, "I'm John Roberts, and this is Kyra Phillips." And he took all the good interviews, leaving me to report the less-important news. I didn't mind playing second fiddle sometimes, but all the time? It was condescending—I wasn't some neophyte reporter with dues to pay. I'd earned more respect than what he was showing me, and I started wondering why I was even there if all he wanted was set dressing.

The producer even had to call us into her office a few times to tell us to get over it or the viewers were going to notice our hostility toward one another.

I didn't know that John's own marriage was falling apart at the time, and that his wife had moved on.

Over time, we began talking before and after the shows. Normal, everyday stuff. We turned some kind of a corner and stopped getting on each other's nerves. He started letting me introduce myself at the top of the show and even shared the "good" interviews.

I was supposed to head back to Atlanta shortly, but then something terrible happened. I got a call from my security company back in Atlanta telling me that the alarm in my foyer was going off.

My neighbor called the cops, then she called me. Her voice was so choked she could barely speak. She sounded like she was hyperventilating. "I'm looking in the front door and I'm looking in the windows and all I see is everything is floating," she said. "Your house is like a swimming pool. You have no ceiling…it's all caved in. Your table is floating…"

I could barely grasp what she was telling me. My house was underwater?

Unthinkable and true. Everything, *everything* was ruined because a toilet pressure valve burst upstairs. There was nothing to salvage. I couldn't go home and see it—I just didn't have it in me. After all the pain and loss of the divorce, I couldn't stand to come face-to-face with that kind of devastation. Some things were replaceable, but others weren't. All of it, gone. Any sense of feeling grounded in Atlanta, gone.

CNN was kind enough to let me stay in New York until I had a place to go back to. The first time I went to see my house was after it had already been gutted. Completely empty, it was as if my entire life had been washed out the front door and there was nothing I could do about it.

"It's like a spiritual cleansing," one of my friends told me.

"Look at it as your opportunity for a real fresh start," said another.

And so I tried. The fact that I had just come back from Baghdad was a blessing; if ever there was a time to let go of my materialism, this was it. Once I got past the initial grief about losing my "stuff," something else took over: a sense of emptiness because that stuff was all I had. I didn't get to have the family I had put off for "someday," and I had a sudden longing for it. I didn't want my life to be measured in place settings, wall hangings and end tables that could all be ruined and taken away from me. There was a permanence missing from my life.

*This is it,* I thought. *It's time to start my life over again and find a better balance.*

I thought about that thing I'd pushed to the back of my mind for so long—having a baby. But was it just a silly fleeting emotion? I dug deeper within myself to ask the tough questions I'd always worried about: Did I have the patience to be a mom? Was I going to want to gouge my ears out at a Wiggles concert, or jump off the nearest balcony at *Disney on Ice*? Did I have it in me to change dirty diapers and sit at the park all afternoon instead of jet-setting all over the world on a moment's notice?

Yes. The answer, finally, was yes. I had done the things I wanted to do in my life, and now I was feeling the pangs that my girlfriends had felt way before I did. I still wanted to be me and to have a career, but I also wanted something deeper in my life. I knew at once that I was ready to have a child.

Of course, fresh on the heels of a divorce, I had picked a pretty strange time to come to this conclusion.

## Can I Have Your Sperm?

It didn't take me long to come up with a plan. I knew that my fertility was in decline just due to my age, so instead of waiting around for the right potential husband to show up, I approached a gay friend of mine named Matt who was visiting me from Los Angeles. He'd been one of my best friends for a long time and he had been encouraging me to get past the divorce and get happy.

"What do you think about being a father? Or fathering my child? Or at least giving me your sperm?" I blurted out without breathing.

"I think it's a fantastic idea!" he said. He knew his odds of being a father any other way were low, and this would give him a chance to know what it was like to be a dad. We lived halfway across the country from one another, so it wouldn't be an everyday parenting experience, but we would visit each other and talk on the phone and share pictures and stories.

"Will you hire a manny?" he asked.

"A what?"

"A gay man to be the nanny. I want the nanny to be someone who would understand me."

"Okay, you got it. Manny it is."

He was totally onboard, his parents were totally onboard and I felt good about the idea that he would be in the child's life. That way, "Daddy" would never be a mystery.

Matt and I went to the clinic I had selected and he donated his sperm, though he emerged from the room looking very distraught.

"What's wrong?" I asked.

"Do you know what they have in those rooms? Hot women porn! What good is that supposed to do me?"

"So what did you do?"

"Turned on my iPod and went into a different world."

Maybe when I told our future child about how Mommy and Daddy decided to make a baby, I'd leave that part out.

Egg retrieval is a much more complex process than sperm donation, so I couldn't have mine done on the spot. I made an appointment to get it started, but then I was sent on assignment and had to postpone it. I felt okay with that, knowing I already had the sperm in the bank and didn't need to rush too much.

Then I got to the business of preparing myself for pregnancy, which was a serious task. In short order, I changed just about everything about my lifestyle. I put away my hookah from Baghdad with all the flavored tobaccos, began eating healthier, added folic acid to my supplement regimen, cut back on caffeine and alcohol, and tried to eliminate any foods with artificial ingredients.

Then there was the emotional side. I went to my first fertility appointment with a girlfriend of mine, and we were both really excited about the possibilities. Then we got inside and noticed tissue boxes everywhere, and couples with sullen faces sitting around the waiting room with their arms crossed.

*Oh,* I thought. *Am I supposed to look sad right now?*

All around me were looks of shame, a sense of failure. And I'd been through it with other friends of mine who'd walked this path. Some of them felt as if they were less womanly because of infertility issues, as if all women are supposed to be fertile and there's something damaged about you if you're not. But I've never wanted to subscribe to that nonsense.

I suspected earlier that I might have a fertility problem because my ex-husband and I had gone so many years without using protection and never conceived. But that didn't make me feel like any less of a woman. It made me feel lucky to be alive in these modern times when infertility doesn't have to mean "the end." It meant I was in for another adventure.

My life hadn't gone as intended. I didn't expect to be single and paying to try to make babies with my gay friend as I approached forty. But I really wasn't sad about it—I didn't allow any stigmas to attach themselves to my psyche. This was a place of hope.

The plan was to harvest my eggs, make embryos with Matt's sperm and then freeze the embryos for a short time while my house in Atlanta was gutted and restored and I could get settled back in after the flood.

And then came Thanksgiving, which changed everything.

# Change of Plans

You're going to think I'm crazy. Or maybe that we had some kind of *Moonlighting* Maddie and David thing going on. But this is what happened: That egotistical anchor John Roberts (who is known as JD) and I actually started enjoying each other's company. I even might have developed the smallest crush on him, and when I moved back to Atlanta, we missed each other.

I was content with my dating life by then; I'd met a number of interesting men and was enjoying the idea of not being tied down to anyone—stopping to smell lots of the flowers, as it were. So when JD called me and said that he'd like to fly in for Thanksgiving and take me to dinner and spend the weekend with me, I was excited, but I didn't get visions of wedding bells dancing in my head. In fact, I was pretty resigned to never share my life, my finances and my space with someone in that manner again. When you get that entwined with someone, you open yourself up to the possibility of a lot of pain, and I wasn't interested in ever being in that kind of pain again, because screw that.

So I agreed to go out with JD, but I was not expecting to fall in love. But I did. Fast. And so did he.

He was nothing like my initial impression of him. We spent Thanksgiving at my best friend's house and I felt so comfortable with him. I quickly learned that this was a very nice man who had just been in a heartbreaking situation at the time. It didn't get ugly the way so many divorces do; JD wanted his ex to be happy, and he wanted their two kids to be happy, so he was doing everything he could to keep his own pain in check. Once it had begun to lift, he was a different person—the real JD.

The real JD was thoughtful and generous and loving, and I could see that this could be my forever guy. But there was an important thing to discuss before it got too serious.

"I want a family," I told him.

He was eleven years older than I was and already had two kids, so I didn't know how he'd react, but he was enthusiastic about it right away. It took me some time and counseling before I was ready to make the commitment—even though I loved JD, I had some trust issues to work through, and I had to make sure he was really over his ex-wife. But we came to a point where we both felt ready, and because I've never really been one for convention, we decided it was more important to try for the baby first . . . there would be plenty of time to get married later.

Poor Matt had exposed himself to hot women porn for nothing.

There came a time when the clinic asked me to decide what to do with the sperm they were saving, and I decided to let it go. I had to FedEx paperwork to Matt so he could give his permission to destroy the sample. It was a really sad moment for both of us; we'd done so much talking and fantasizing about our future child—or children— together, and at times he'd been even more eager about it than I was.

I hated that I was now cutting him out of the equation. It just didn't make sense anymore if I was committing to a new relationship.

But there was still one more surprise for me:

"I had a vasectomy," JD said.

Oh.

Well, in that case, it was a good thing I'd already started the process at a clinic! Given my age and the fact that I'd never gotten pregnant before, we probably would have wound up there anyway, but now it was a definite. There was no way I'd get pregnant naturally.

The doctors could have performed a vasectomy reversal on JD, but that's a difficult procedure that doesn't have an immediate effect: It can take one to two years before everything is functioning normally again and, depending on a bunch of factors, like how long ago the procedure was done, it might not even work. My eggs weren't about to sit around waiting for one to two years to see if it was successful. So there was another option: The doctors could do microsurgery on JD to retrieve sperm from the testes without having to reverse the vasectomy. They said it would be less invasive, with a shorter recovery time and a better chance of success. Was this a trick question? *Sign us the heck up.*

So there I sat with my aging eggs in this office full of depressed people, and all I could think about was how cool it was that this pregnancy thing might happen for me really soon. I wasn't sure exactly how or when, but I felt really good about the whole possibility. *Hey, thanks, science.*

I'll tell you more about the process when we get to the chapters about infertility treatments in Part 2 of this book, but I won't keep you in suspense about the ending: We ended up working with Jamie and having beautiful twins. The process changed me, and it was so important to have a doctor like Jamie on my side. He became so much more than just a doctor to me: He was a trusted confidante, therapist, supporter and friend. There's a lot to process when it comes to fertility treatments and having the right doctor can make a huge difference in how you get through it all emotionally.

Being a parent is even better than I ever hoped it would be. I hope it'll be like that for you, too.

# Jamie's Story

Since I was very young, I always thought I'd go into medicine or science. I was a tinkerer and I loved to discover and invent, and also had a passion for health. As it turned out, I never really had to make a choice between the two fields.

In college, I majored in biology and chemistry. Rather than go straight into either research or medicine afterwards, I got into an MD-PhD program that allowed me to do both and decide later. The most logical progression for me was to go into cancer research, but I wasn't so sure I liked the idea of sitting in a lab without much human interaction.

*Maybe I could be a pediatrician*, I thought. I always liked kids, and I had a good sense of empathy. That would appeal to one part of my personality, but it still left out the part of me that wanted to discover and break new ground.

I graduated from medical school right around the time when things were just heating up in reproductive medicine. The first in vitro fertilization (IVF) baby had just been born and it seemed that this was a field with a lot of possibility for growth and change. At the last minute, I changed tracks and decided to specialize in obstetrics and gynecology (OB/GYN).

I'd done some study in the field and liked that we were now able to perform amniocentesis to do genetic testing on an unborn baby—

but what I found more interesting was the possibility of doing genetic testing even before there was a pregnancy: testing embryos before implanting them into the mother. Doing so could help us avoid all kinds of diseases and serious health conditions, as well as lowering miscarriage rates. I had seen that some researchers were doing this on animals, so that's what I focused on during my fellowship and what led me to become a fertility specialist.

Translational research has been my forte; I like translating research into real-life applications as opposed to just increasing the body of knowledge on a topic. It's more interesting to me to help enact changes in the way we practice medicine, so that's what I set out to do. I helped to make major advances in embryonic genetic testing and egg freezing and thawing techniques while also seeing patients regularly.

What surprised me the most about the field was that it didn't just require me to be a fertility expert but also a de facto psychologist. There is so much emotion within the walls of a fertility clinic. There are spoken and unspoken fears, heartbreaks when the process doesn't go right or ends badly, tensions in relationships, overwhelming amounts of stress and anxiety, and, of course, overwhelming amounts of joy on the other end of the spectrum. It would never be worth it without that payoff; I do have many sleepless nights and times when the pressure of carrying so many people's dreams in my hands follows me home. I need to decompress from it all each night because every day is full of such high stakes—we're literally creating life, and the timing and the details count.

## Favorite Successes

Back when I was still doing preimplantation genetic diagnostic testing on animals, a savvy woman who read medical journals learned about my work and sought me out.

"I'd like to be your first human test subject," she said. She was a known carrier of hemophilia, which meant that any male babies she'd have would be at risk. Girls may carry the disease, but they are not normally symptomatic. Therefore, this woman felt that the most responsible thing she could do would be to ensure that she had a girl.

We could do that by doing an egg retrieval, combining eggs with her husband's sperm and then testing the embryos to see which ones had female chromosomes. That's just what we did, and she became the very first preimplantation genetic diagnostic success story in the United States.

Fourteen years later, I was walking by a restaurant when I had a pang of recognition of a couple sitting at a table with their daughter. I wasn't sure why I knew them, but I was sure I'd seen them before.

"Dr. Grifo!" the woman said, and my memory came into focus. It was her. Sitting a few feet away from me was this fourteen-year-old "baby" that had once lived in a little petri dish in my lab. I love those moments.

One of my earliest patients, a single woman who used donor sperm, visited me in a more planned fashion. She lived far away and wanted to know if it would be okay to bring her daughter on a trip to meet "the man who helped." I loved how her mother handled the story and how graceful and respectful her daughter was of the way she'd been brought up. She was about to enter college, and I asked her, "What was it like going through school without a dad when most of your classmates had a father in their lives?"

"You know what?" she asked. "I'm just lucky I got the mom I got."

It impressed me that she didn't feel cheated; instead, she appreciated the choice her mother had made for her. It reinforced my belief that what matters is how much you are loved in this world, not the method by which you came into it.

Many of the "firsts"—the first successful IVF, the first baby born after egg freezing—have special meaning to me. But there are so many others that have special places in my heart, too. People have traveled from all over the world to come to our clinic and trust us with their most important dreams. It's an honor to get to be a part of their stories and know that they might not have had the families they hoped for without our help.

My best teacher was my own fertility journey with my wife. We were unable to conceive on our own and so we turned to IVF. I don't believe you can ever really understand something until you've been through it yourself, and this gave me new insights into my patients. We were confronted with the same fears that everyone else was:

*What if this doesn't work?*

*What will my life look like if I never have the children I want?*

My wife took it very well, but it was not an easy process for us, nor did we get an unfair advantage with our success rate. It was a protracted journey with twists and turns, but, in the end, we have our family. That's a pretty great success.

## Life as a Fertility Doctor

You see and hear a lot of crazy things as a fertility doctor. No two situations are alike, even though some of the underlying emotions and fears are the same. And some individual situations evolve over time. What happens when a couple undergoing IVF splits up? What do they do with the embryos? Most of the time the couple agree to discard them, but what if one person still wants to go forward with it and the other doesn't? You can't make someone a parent who no longer wants to be one, so we require the consent of both parties to go forward—which sometimes leads to more drama in the workplace than you'd imagine.

Sometimes, couples also change their minds about how far they're willing to go and what options they're willing to try. Just about every couple will say up front that they would never, ever consider using an egg donor, yet when they run out of other options, some decide to go for it. Having a baby they can love becomes more important than having a baby with matching DNA.

And then there are the people who get angry when it turns out that I can't perform magic. Fertility medicine is a wonderful field that's come a long way, but it will never be 100 percent effective. It doesn't work for everyone, and that makes some people look for a place to point the blame. I'm a handy target. Sometimes people get mad if I can't get them pregnant, and sometimes people get mad if I do! I even had one woman complain bitterly because I had told her that her odds of success were low, based on her age (they were), but we implanted two embryos and she wound up pregnant with twins. Despite the positive result, she was upset that I hurt her feelings by telling her that her chances were low.

But there are so many more good outcomes than bad. Some of the couples who don't succeed with IVF still thank me afterwards because they know they've given it their best shot and can move on with their other options. But more often, I get thanked in the form of holiday cards, letters and visits from the children who started as embryos in our clinic. Many of them are now graduating from college, and I wonder what they'll do with their lives. Will there be any Olympians among them? Nobel Prize winners? Future presidents? I don't know, but I do know this: What I do for a living is very cool and very rewarding. I have a hand in changing the world every day, and that makes me feel terrific. I'm just one part of the machine, but I love getting to be a part of it.

# Introduction:

## Fertility for Life

## By Kyra Phillips

Lots of women will tell you that being a mom is the greatest thing on the planet. I'm going to let you in on a secret: It is…if you're ready for it.

I always knew I wanted to have a family *someday*, but it took until my late thirties before it felt like *someday* had come. I knew my fertility wasn't going to last forever, but I didn't know there was anything I could do about it. I just hoped my "window" hadn't passed me by. Now I know there were things I could have done to take control of my fertility.

We know that the best *biological* time to have a baby is in our teens and twenties, but that's not usually the most *practical* time. As we get older, some of us panic if we're not married, financially stable and ready to have kids. One option is to rush ahead anyway, to meet a guy and make a baby because we worry it's getting too late. That, my friend, is the stupid option.

I didn't know that there was a better option until I met Dr. Jamie Grifo.

When my husband and I were trying to conceive, I began working with Jamie, one of the country's foremost fertility doctors. As the father of five kids and program director of the NYU Fertility Center—and as someone who had gone through the infertility process himself—Jamie understood the journey from all angles. His insight, expertise and sensitivity to my situation helped me beyond measure. It was not an easy road going through in vitro fertilization (IVF) and experiencing several miscarriages. Jamie taught me how I could improve my odds of conceiving, and things I should have been doing (and not doing) in my twenties and thirties to prepare for my future in babymaking.

Had I known earlier the things Jamie told me, I would have made different choices that might have made my road a lot easier and saved me some heartache. He taught me about egg freezing and the lightning-speed changes in that field—what used to be a long-shot hope is now a very solid possibility for putting your fertility "on ice" until you're ready. He taught me about how the choices I made with regard to things like drinking, smoking, drugs, sex, food, exercise, supplements and gynecological exams could have affected my fertility.

And I'd like to tell you it was all my husband, but Jamie Grifo is the man who got me pregnant. So I listen to him.

Once I got through the process and had my wonderful twins, I said to Jamie, "Women should know about this stuff a lot sooner!" It didn't seem right that the first time anyone had taught me how to take care of my fertility was when I was sitting in a fertility clinic at forty years old. They don't teach us this stuff in high school health class, and our mothers don't know enough about it to teach us, either. There are books out there about what to do when you already know you're infertile, but what about before that point? What about trying to preserve your fertility *before* it sneaks out the window and runs away?

And so Jamie and I decided we should write a book—the book I wish I'd had when I was in my twenties. We wanted to get the word out that there are things within your control, and that the time to start thinking about your fertility is immediately, even if you're not planning to have any babies for another ten years. The things you do today could have permanent consequences, so it's important to know as much as you can about the facts and the myths of how to preserve your fertility.

In this book, Jamie and I are going to tell you about what I went through and what you can learn from it. We're also going to separate fact from fiction about fertility aids and techniques. Whether you're twenty or forty, there's still a lot within your control.

Here are some things we'll cover:

- What to ask your gynecologist at every annual exam, even long before you're ready to have a baby
- Whether dropping acid once in college...okay, twice... is going to screw up your eggs
- How smoking affects your fertility
- What gynecological conditions you may not know you have, and how to fix them
- Which STIs (sexually transmitted infections) and STDs (sexually transmitted diseases) can ruin your chances of having a baby
- Whether or not infertility—or great fertility—is genetic
- When you need to stop partying
- What your weight has to do with your fertility
- How men can preserve or screw up their fertility, too

- What fertility treatments are like, and what your options
  are if you need them

Throughout the book, there will be some places where I'll tell pieces of my own story, and places where Jamie will tell about things he's experienced in the fertility lab. Otherwise, the book is written in our voice together.

Thanks for letting us come along on your fertility journey; we hope you'll learn a lot and have a few laughs at my expense along the way. Wait until you get to the hemorrhoid story...

# Part One

# Preserving Your Fertility

# Chapter 1
# Baby, Maybe

## Delaying Motherhood

In 1970, the average age for a first-time mother was twenty-one, and about 36 percent of all births were to women who were teenagers or younger. It's only recently that we associate teen parenting with poor choices; it was once the norm. Now, keep in mind that the average age for marriage back then was twenty, and you'll see quickly why the babies tended to arrive a year later.

But a lot has happened since the Baby Boomer generation grew up—for one thing, the divorce rate skyrocketed, with Baby Boomers often explaining, "We were too young." For another thing, the workplace became much more competitive as more jobs began requiring college degrees and advanced degrees. Kids were no longer graduating from high school, getting married and finding good-paying work to support their families on one person's salary without any postsecondary education.

Today, 66 percent of young adults in the United States go to college, and about 10 percent go on to graduate school. Then they enter the workforce, where the norm is working your way up from low-level jobs to the position you're aiming for over the course of several years—which could mean into your thirties and forties. Another big change is that women are no longer primarily housewives; they are closing the gap and pulling in nearly half the household income. Women have careers, not just little things they do on the side to make some extra money while their husbands are expected to be the main breadwinners. They even have actual career ambitions, where they now get to have this revolutionary notion that their work can be meaningful and that they're not built solely to be babymaking machines.

We also have easier access to birth control, and less stigma about using it, so we're able to plan more carefully when we want to have kids. Ninety-eight percent of Catholic women say they've used birth control at some point, despite the church's official position against it.

It is in part because of all this that the average ages for both marriage and motherhood has been on the rise. Currently, the average first-time bride in the United States is twenty-seven and the average first-time groom is twenty-nine. People are waiting until they finish school and get more established in their careers before they decide to get married and make babies—not always in that order. In fact, now 48 percent of all babies born in the United States are to unmarried moms! That's right—nearly half. In fact, the only women who follow the script of our ancestors more often than not (marriage first, then babies) are college graduates, who tend to have their first babies at age thirty. Women who don't go to college or don't finish tend to have babies first, then get married a couple of years later, if at all.

And that's the other major change: Marriage is no longer a foregone conclusion. Whereas in 1920, ninety-two women got married each year out of every thousand single women of marrying age, in 2013, that number was cut to a third—thirty-one women per thousand and still dropping. Not everyone has dreams of a big wedding celebration; we're increasingly a society where marriage is optional, not expected. The figures vary based on race as well: Only 26 percent of African-American women are now married, compared to 45 percent of Hispanic women and 51 percent of Caucasian women.[1]

The thing about babymaking is that you can make all the plans you want, but you can't force the right time. You can't even force the right time when Mother Nature wants it to happen. She's all about the teens and early twenties, but how many people do you know who really have their act together by then? Most of us are busy learning how much alcohol we can consume before we start finding the nearest lamppost attractive, what we're supposed to do with our lives now that we're "grown up" and where we're supposed to live now that we can pay our own rent.

Some of us get it right on the first try and some don't. Our friend Jenna got married at twenty-seven, was pregnant right "on schedule" at age thirty and she planned to have two more kids pretty quickly. Her dream was to have three kids, two years apart apiece. But her marriage failed, and she was left wondering how long she could hang onto her fertility. Would the right guy come along quickly? Or would it be too late for more kids by the time he showed up? And how could she stack the deck in her favor?

Or consider Diem Brown, whose dreams of having kids of her own were nearly obliterated when she got ovarian cancer at age twenty-three and a recurrence seven years later. She needed to have her ovaries removed, but she couldn't force herself to have a baby before that point. If she wanted to have her own biological children, the only possible way for her to do it was to freeze her eggs before the surgeon removed the remaining piece of her ovary, so that's what she did. It's amazing that she had that opportunity.

But the less dire circumstances are more typical—what if you're just a twentysomething woman who knows she wants to have kids someday, but isn't in a life circumstance to have them yet? So many factors come into play before you make the decision to have a baby, and while there may never be a "perfect" time, there are certainly some key factors that go into most people's choices—economic stability and relationship stability topping the list, plus things like emotional readiness and maturity, career flexibility and a support system. You don't want to run out and get pregnant before you have your act together just because you're afraid your eggs are shriveling up.

Don't pressure yourself. Yes, there is a biological clock, and, yes, it will eventually run out for everyone. But there are things you can do to keep that clock ticking until its last possible second, and that's what we're here to help you with.

## Your Biological Clock

Unfortunately, when your egg supply runs out (or at least out of good-quality eggs), that's it. *C'est la vie.* You have to start thinking about your options aside from having children who are biologically yours (and there are, of course, many options for that—adopting, fostering, having an egg donor or using a surrogate). But what often happens is that long before your egg supply runs out, the eggs get depleted or damaged along the way, leading to decreased fertility—so women are behind the 8-ball before they even think about having a child. And in most cases, it happens without any advance notice. Your ovaries don't text you to say, "Egg supply approaching critical—shutdown imminent—make baby now!"

You can't add time to the biological clock you were born with, but what you can do is make sure that you get every minute that you're entitled to, and not lose time because of bad choices you've made, risks you didn't know you were taking or things you didn't take care of when you should have. Fertility is one of those things that no one teaches you about until you're already having problems.

One of the most frustrating things about fertility is that just as you're ready to launch into your amazing and exciting life, your ovaries are already planning for retirement. Believe it or not, your fertility begins to decline in your twenties, then continues on a steady downward slope all through your thirties. While infertility can be present at any age, thirty-five has been tossed around as the edge of that fertility cliff. We don't agree with that number; forty is the more accurate danger zone. Your chances of conceiving naturally even in your late thirties are still good, but at forty, that changes. Every two years after age forty, your fertility is cut in half again. The trajectory looks like this:

## Pregnancy Rates within One Year

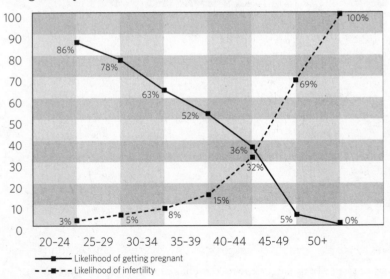

Source: Andrew Toledo, MD, Reproductive Biology Associates

What's more troubling is that these numbers merely reflect the likelihood of *getting pregnant*. Getting all the way to having an actual crying, spitting up and pooping bundle of wake-me-up-every-two-hours-when-I'm-exhausted-beyond-belief adds another whole degree of uncertainty.

We all know about the exceptions—your mother's neighbor's cousin's best friend who thought she was in menopause and instead had her "surprise baby" at forty-nine, or a fifty-two-year-old woman in China who didn't even know she was pregnant until she was rushed to the hospital with what she thought was appendicitis and turned out to be active labor. Yeah, it happens, but it's crazy rare, and that's exactly why we hear about it. It's surprising news.

## Kyra Says . . .

I knew that my fertility was in decline, but I didn't think that was a big deal as long as I could afford fertility treatments. I thought, "I'll just wait until I'm ready, then have the doc whip up an egg and sperm white soufflé, prick it and pat it and mark it with a 'B' and put it in the oven for baby and me!" Was I naive.

Knowing what I know now, I would have done things differently. And it wouldn't have been to rush into having a baby at an earlier age. I would have prepared better for the time when I was ready.

Be aware that even in your peak fertility years, it can take quite some time to get pregnant. In fact, the chance of conception per month is about 10 percent and it takes thirteen months of trying for 100 percent of fertile twenty-five-year-old women to get pregnant. Not only is it much less likely for you to conceive naturally each cycle once you hit your late thirties, but it's also less likely for in vitro fertilization (IVF) to work as you get older. So your odds of conceiving using IVF are a lot better than your odds without, but it's far from a guarantee. From 2003 to 2011, the New York University (NYU) Fertility Center charted its success rates for each cycle of IVF, and here's what they looked like:

| MATERNAL AGE | LIVE BIRTH PER EMBRYO TRANSFER |
|---|---|
| Under 30 | 58% |
| 30 | 59% |
| 31 | 53% |
| 32 | 52% |
| 33 | 46% |
| 34 | 51% |
| 35 | 46% |
| 36 | 43% |
| 37 | 43% |
| 38 | 39% |
| 39 | 32% |
| 40 | 28% |
| 41 | 26% |
| 42 | 14% |
| 43 | 13% |
| 44 | 6% |
| 45 and up | 1% |

So basically, if you're thirty-two or under and have experienced infertility, the odds are in your favor that you'll have a pregnancy ending in a live birth with just a single IVF cycle. You've got a pretty good chance of hitting a home run your first time at bat. But at age forty-two, your odds are just 14 percent of having that same procedure work on the first try. And remember—IVF isn't cheap.

# Egg Quality

They don't teach you about fertility in health class—well, beyond just telling you to keep your legs closed and not get pregnant. But there are things we should all know—things we don't talk about enough as a society—so we can make informed decisions about our bodies and our futures and so we can learn how to exert some control over Mother Nature.

One thing to know is that it's not just a matter of running out of eggs. You can have the best fertility doctor in the world and still not succeed if your eggs are all shot.

So what's a "good-quality" egg?

The first test is its chromosomes: Most egg defects are chromosomal abnormalities. People are supposed to have twenty-three pairs of chromosomes, and these chromosomes store DNA. There are some chromosomal abnormalities that cause birth disorders such as Down syndrome, which results from all or part of an extra copy of chromosome 21. Some abnormalities are worse and can cause certain death of the child if a pregnancy is carried to term. Chromosomal abnormalities in embryos are also responsible for 80 percent of miscarriages.

That's why insensitive people may say that miscarriages are "God's way" or "nature's way" of rooting out babies who would have been born with birth defects. While it's clear that most of the embryos that are miscarried would have had significant disabilities or birth defects, each case is different, and doctors don't always know why a chromosomal abnormality causes a miscarriage.

In our twenties and early thirties, most of our eggs should be of good quality with normal chromosomes, but as we age, not only are there fewer eggs left, but those eggs are more and more likely to have chromosomal damage, due to both aging and outside factors that we'll get into later in the book. And you can't tell by looking at someone what her fertility is like. There's this fantasy notion that if you look younger than you are, then you're probably totally fertile. As if because your skin looks youthful, you're probably all youthful inside, too. False. You can't fool those reproductive organs. They're in there getting all geriatric even as you walk around looking hot in a minidress.

Energy production also declines as we age. It takes a lot of energy to make a baby! And not just in that way, you cheeky person, you. For about twelve hours after conception, the fertilized egg is still just one cell, but all hell is about to break loose. Inside our eggs, the mitochondria produce energy to divide the cells and chromosomes. If the conception is successful, then the cell divides over and over until it's a raspberry-shaped blastocyst consisting of hundreds of cells, which then enters the uterus and tries to implant itself into the endometrium—the lining of the uterus. But the problem is that sometimes the mitochondria punk out. Especially as we age, our mitochondria can run out of steam before finishing the job. They can start the marathon looking strong, but end up weaving back and forth and calling for a stretcher before the end of the first mile.

So many things have to go just right for a pregnancy to result in a healthy baby that it's amazing it happens as often as it does!

And, yes, each of us has a "best-before" date on our ovaries. But as we've been saying, there are things we can do to make sure that day doesn't come any sooner than it has to, and that's what we're going to discuss, starting . . . right now!

# Chapter 2
# Sex and Fertility

Aside from aging, sexually transmitted diseases (STDs) are the single greatest threat to a woman's fertility. (It's a threat to men's fertility, too, but less so.) Almost any STD can cause damage to the reproductive tract, though some are worse than others in that regard. It's within your control to take charge of this aspect of your fertility, so be smart about it.

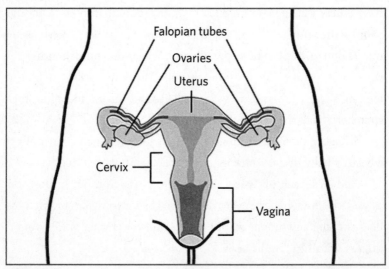

Source: Centers for Disease Control and Prevention

# How You Get Knocked Up

To understand how various things can harm your fertility, you first need to know how your body gets pregnant. Let's take a quick tour of your reproductive system.

Unlike men, who have the ability to make sperm throughout their lives, women are born with all the eggs they'll ever have. The crazy part is this: When you're a twenty-week-old fetus developing in your mother's womb, you have about 7 million eggs. By the time you're born, you have only 1–2 million eggs left. No one knows why; it's a biologically weird process called atresia, where your eggs die off and are absorbed by the immune system. The eggs are immature and can't be used to produce babies until they go through a growth process.

But atresia keeps on happening, and by the time you hit puberty, you're down to just 600,000 of your original 7 million eggs. Every menstrual cycle, you lose about a thousand more eggs. By age thirty, you've lost 87 percent of your eggs, and by forty, you've lost 97 percent of your eggs. It's a really inefficient process, but it's similar to the plant world: Farmers have to plant a lot of seeds to get one healthy plant. Seeds have just a 10 percent germination rate, on average.

## Jamie Says . . .

I went to a farmstand about ten years ago, and the elderly farmer noticed my "MD" license plates.

"What kind of doc are you?" he asked.

"I'm a fertility specialist," I said.

"One of those embryo guys?"

"Yes."

continued on page 14

"So you're a farmer like me."

"Sir? What do you mean?"

"I plant seeds . . . you plant seeds." Then he smiled and said, "But I bet I'm better than you."

"Excuse me?"

He led me to the back of the barn, where there were ten beautiful plants lined up.

"How many seeds do you think I had to plant to get those beauties?"

I thought hard, all the way back to my college botany classes, where I learned that the germination rate of seeds is 10 percent.

"Man, Doc, you're good. But I'm still better than you."

I had to laugh because he was right—the literature from our lab revealed that about 5 percent of eggs make babies. Whether in the lab or at home in bed, not all eggs are good eggs and there's only so much we can control. Much like farmers, we are dealing with a highly imperfect "germination rate," and there's no point in stressing out about trying to get every egg to be "the one" that will make a healthy baby. They're just not all qualified for that role.

Your eggs are in two almond-size-and-shaped ovaries on either side of your pelvis. Each month, provided things are working right, a bunch of immature eggs start growing inside sacs (called follicles) in your ovaries. Then one of those eggs "hatches," leaving the follicle, and the ovary releases it about two weeks before your period starts. That's ovulation. Over the course of your life, only about four hundred eggs will ever be released. These are your four hundred possibilities of getting pregnant.

After ovulation, the egg ventures out of the follicle and gets sucked up into the fallopian tubes (which aren't directly connected to the ovary, but are nearby in the abdominal cavity). The fallopian tubes are three to six inches long and have fingerlike tentacles at the end that help push the egg through. If sperm come swimming in through the cervix, they try to meet up with the egg in the fallopian tube, which has the perfect environment for fertilization—nutrition and sweet, sweet Al Green music playing in the background.

About 75 million sperm at a time take this journey together (that's not a typo), but most of them die before they make it to the egg. Some die off right away because of the acidic environment of the vagina, others get stuck in the folds of the cervix and some get attacked by the woman's immune system because it mistakes the sperm for an invader. About half of the survivors don't stop to ask directions and end up in the wrong fallopian tube—the one without a waiting egg. The remaining sperm have to then make it past the cilia that line the fallopian tubes (where some of them get stuck and die) and into the sperm receptors in the egg's membrane, called the zona pellucida. Those extreme athletes get hyperactive at the end so they can swim with greater strength and faster now that the target is in sight.

They smash their little sperm noggins against the egg's membrane and try to penetrate it. Once one of them makes it through that final barrier, the egg is officially fertilized and shuts down the membrane's gates, making sure that no other sperm can get in. She's already spoken for.

The fertilized egg then starts dividing right away and takes a leisurely stroll through the snug confines of the fallopian tube and into the vastness of the uterus, where it tries to attach, or implant. If it manages to burrow down into the fluffy blood-rich tissue of the endometrium (think soft red velvet sheets here) then the egg can start growing from an embryo into a baby.

The biggest threat to this magical process is if a sexually transmitted infection (STI) causes damage to some part of a woman's reproductive system and prevents ovulation, fertilization, implantation or the ability to carry a baby to full term.

So here's where you have to be smart.

# STIs and Fertility

When you're out there dating and having fun, childbearing may not be looming large in your consciousness—but the guy you sleep with today could end up screwing up your chance to have a baby with Mr. Right ten years down the road.

Chances are good that you've had it drummed into your head that "safer sex" practices are good and STIs/STDs are bad, but here's something we can tell you: All this talking we've done as a society about safer sex hasn't solved the problem. Each year, there are 20 million new diagnoses of sexually transmitted diseases, and nearly half of them are people in the fifteen- to twenty-four-year-old age bracket. I don't have to tell you that some of those diseases are incurable, meaning that the not-very-good sex a seventeen-year-old had while her parents were out can result in bumps and rashes and much worse things *for the rest of her life.* Of course, it can also affect all her future sex partners and their partners, and some can even affect her children before they're born.

You'd think that would be enough to ensure that every sexually active teen and young adult in the country would have a serious stock of condoms on hand, but when the Centers for Disease Control and Prevention (CDC) surveyed high school students in 2011, they found that among kids who acknowledged they were sexually active in the last three months (which was about 34 percent of all the kids they surveyed), nearly 40 percent *did not use a condom* the last time they had sex.

Why are young people not using condoms? Well, there are a bunch of reasons. They're embarrassed to buy them, they don't have money, they're afraid to ask their partner to use one, they think it's a sign of mistrust, they think it won't feel as good, they're not expecting to have sex and it "just happens"...

But these sorts of excuses and rationalizations are not limited to students. People of all ages find reasons not to do the responsible thing. In fact, men over fifty are the worst group of all when it comes to condom use—they use a condom only 28 percent of the time when they're having casual sex, according to the National Survey of Sexual Health and Behavior, a recent major study by Indiana University.

People of all ages are only semi-reliably using condoms, and they're out there getting infected with STIs without even knowing it because symptoms (a) may take a long time to show up, (b) may be so mild that they're barely noticeable or attributed to other things, such as a cold or flu, and (c) may not show up at all. Yes, you can definitely have an STI and never show any outward signs of it—but it can still damage your reproductive system.

A study among college students showed that 62 percent of them believed they would know if someone had an STI "just by looking," which is a dangerous myth. There are few STIs and STDs that have visible symptoms. Most are invisible to the eye.

We know a guy who said he didn't have to worry about condoms because he dated only "nice, clean girls." He got herpes. He was lucky that's all he got.

# Which Ones Can Mess with You

Certain STDs are a lot more likely to cause serious fertility damage than others. Here are the worst offenders.

## Chlamydia

Chlamydia is the most common STD that is caused by bacteria, and yet most people who are infected don't even know it. That's why it's called the "silent STD." About 1.5 million cases are reported annually, and researchers at the CDC think twice as many people are walking around with it undiagnosed. The number of cases has more than doubled in the past ten years, and it's most common in women aged fifteen to twenty-four. At least one in fifteen women in that age group has it, so even if you don't have it, you can be pretty well assured that at least one of your girlfriends does.

If you do get any symptoms, they're probably mild or you can explain them away by other things. Symptoms include vaginal discharge (sometimes with an odor), a burning sensation when peeing, bleeding in between your periods, lower back pain, fever, pain during sex, rectal pain and rectal discharge and/or bleeding. Men might also get swelling or discharge from the penis. But if you're like the 75 percent of women with no symptoms, you won't notice anything at all, and the bacteria will start infecting your cervix or urethra. If it's not treated, that's when things get more serious: It can move upward through your reproductive tract and can get into your uterus and fallopian tubes. About 40 percent of cases result in pelvic inflammatory disease (PID). Fortunately, this doesn't happen in every case, but it is unclear why some women are luckier than others; just being healthy does not protect you.

PID can cause pelvic and abdominal pain but, just like chlamydia itself, it can also be symptomless. And it can cause permanent infertility (more on why later) and raise the risk of ectopic pregnancy (pregnancy that happens outside the uterus and has to be terminated or else you could die).

Because chlamydia is so common in the younger age group, the CDC recommends that everyone under age twenty-five who is sexually active get tested for it once a year. After that point, you should get tested again whenever you have a new sex partner. It's a simple test—you just have to pee in a cup or get swabbed, and insurance usually covers it. You can also get it done for free or inexpensively at a clinic.

Chlamydia is spread by any kind of sexual contact: vaginal, anal or oral. It's a lot easier to get it by vaginal or anal sex, but you can get it while giving a blow job (and he can get it from your mouth while you're giving him this—undoubtedly awesome—blow job) and it can infect your throat. A man doesn't need to ejaculate to infect you. Use a condom or a dental dam during oral sex unless you're in a monogamous relationship where both partners have been tested for all the common STDs.

In men, chlamydia symptoms include burning, itching and discharge from the penis; and pain and swelling in the testicles. It can also lead to infertility in men. A Swedish study of 244 infertile couples and 244 pregnant couples found that couples where the male tested positive for chlamydia antibodies were one-third less likely to achieve pregnancy.[1]

Chlamydia can also be passed to the baby if you're infected while pregnant; newborns with chlamydia often get eye infections and pneumonia within three to six weeks of birth.

Now for the good news! It's very easily treatable, but you have to catch it early. Just a course of antibiotics will knock it out, and you have to avoid sex for only a week. There's a significant risk of reinfection, though, especially if your partner doesn't get treated at the same time. He doesn't have to have any symptoms; he should be treated no matter what if you're infected. Each time you get reinfected, you're putting your fertility at greater and greater risk—it is cumulative—so consider the first infection your wake-up call. Always use condoms and make sure your partners have been tested and treated.

If you've already had it, should you freak out? No—there are plenty of women who have had it and still get pregnant without trouble.

It mostly depends on how bad the infection got, how long you had it and whether or not it progressed to PID. If it did, you may have some hurdles, but they're typically not insurmountable.

## Jamie Says . . .

Teresa* came to my clinic at age thirty-three trying to figure out why she couldn't get pregnant. She and her partner had been trying for more than a year. I saw on a laparoscopy that her tubes were blocked and she had Fitz-Hugh-Curtis syndrome, inflammation in the tissues that line the whole abdominal cavity and characteristically exhibits bands of adhesions between the liver and diaphragm, which are surprisingly asymptomatic. Adhesions are scarlike tissues that connect surfaces inside the body that are not meant to be connected. They're not an uncommon complication of pelvic inflammatory disease (which may follow chlamydia or a gonorrhea infection, most commonly).

Teresa had obviously had such a bad infection that it caused these terrible adhesions, and her tubes were filled with fluid. All that damage was done by a silent infection she never knew she had. The infection traveled up her cervix and into her fallopian tubes, and the damage came from her body going into overdrive to kill the bacteria, creating scar tissue all over her reproductive tract and ruining her tubes.

Tests for chlamydia and gonorrhea were both negative because her body had cleared the infection long ago, but she now had permanent scars to show for it.

Most likely, it had happened in her twenties. She mentioned that she'd had some abdominal discomfort then and had been

---

* All names of patients have been changed.

treated for irritable bowel syndrome, but it's likely that the discomfort was really a result of this untreated infection that led to complications. How could she have guessed, though, that abdominal pains were related to an STD?

She'd only had two partners, she told me, and now she was facing the truth that her only feasible option for pregnancy would be removing her tubes and doing IVF. It was frustrating to know that early diagnosis and treatment likely would have prevented the infection from traveling any further and could have saved her fertility.

## Gonorrhea

The second STD that most commonly threatens fertility is gonorrhea, which is sometimes confused with chlamydia. It is also spread by any kind of sexual contact (vaginal, anal or oral) and a man doesn't need to ejaculate to infect you.

As with chlamydia, women with gonorrhea often have no symptoms. If you do get symptoms, they usually show up within about ten days of infection, and can include pain or burning when peeing, unusual vaginal discharge, bleeding between periods, heavy periods and pain during sex. Men may notice white, yellow or green discharge from the penis and painful or swollen testicles. Or they might not.

And also, as with chlamydia, the main problem is that when it's untreated, it can travel to your uterus and cause PID. Basically, you've got to catch your symptomless STD early if you want to ensure that it doesn't do permanent damage.

The news about treatment for gonorrhea is iffy. It used to be that it was just as easy to treat as chlamydia was—just take a single dose of antibiotics and you're good to go. But now there are lots of antibiotic-resistant strains of the disease and doctors are running out of options. In the 1970s and '80s, they treated it with penicillin and tetracyclines, but it developed resistance to those drugs. Then doctors began using fluoroquinolones (ciprofloxacin, ofloxacin or levofloxacin), but by the early 2000s, these became resistant, too, and the CDC recommended that doctors stop prescribing that class of drugs for gonorrhea and PID because there was staggering proof that it wasn't working anymore—the bacteria had outsmarted the drug.

There was just one class of drugs left to treat gonorrhea: the cephalosporins. Primarily, doctors prescribed cefixime, brand name Suprax. But in 2012, the CDC issued a giant warning to doctors: Stop prescribing the oral antibiotic, because it's happening all over again— gonorrhea is becoming resistant to it, we're afraid the disease will soon be resistant to the whole class of drugs and we're at the end of our rope. The only recommended treatment now for the disease is an injectable antibiotic in the same class, ceftriaxone. It can be given along with one of two other oral antibiotics (azithromycin or doxycycline) to boost effectiveness. But basically, we know we're about to be in real trouble. History shows us that gonorrhea is going to find a way around this drug, too, and then there's nothing else that's been proven effective. We're just trying to buy time until someone comes up with another treatment that works . . . and if we don't find another treatment in time, then we're going to have a whole lot of people with raging gonorrhea.

But there are some problems with offering only injectable medication, too. First, some people just won't do it because they hate needles, and second, it messes up what doctors often do for the infected person's partners: To make sure the partner gets treated, the doctor would just call in a prescription of the same antibiotic for that person. Now the partner needs to come in separately and get an injection, too, which may not happen if the person isn't feeling any symptoms and thinks that means there's no problem.

Then that infected partner goes on to infect someone else, or reinfects the person who was already treated. And so on, and so on. It also leaves you more susceptible to other STDs, particularly HIV.

As of now, the treatments are still working in more than 90 percent of cases—and in the cases where the antibiotic fails, a double dose of it in the second round usually knocks it out. But it's critical to get tested and get treated early if you find out you've been infected, because there is no medication to reverse the damage it does to your reproductive tract. You can be left permanently infertile, even if the gonorrhea is successfully treated.

It can also be passed to your newborn during the delivery process, with devastating consequences.

# HPV

There has been some controversy about whether or not the very common STD HPV (human papillomavirus) causes infertility. The short answer is that it doesn't. A small study done in 2006 showed a significantly lower success rate for women with HPV who went for IVF treatments, but a bunch of other studies thereafter showed that there was no statistical difference between women with or without HPV. So don't freak if you've had it. However, we know for certain that both the complications of and the treatments for HPV can contribute to infertility.

Some facts: HPV is so common that 80 percent of women will have it at some point in their lives, even if you have just one partner for years and years and he isn't cheating on you. Normally, it goes away on its own within a few years and you won't even know you ever had it. But there are more than forty types of HPV and they cause different problems: Some cause genital warts, for instance (you'll probably know if you have those!), some cause warts in the throat and some cause cervical cancer (and other types of cancers, but less commonly).

And because the virus lives on the skin, you can get HPV from any intimate contact, even if you're using a condom, because it can be in the areas around a guy's penis and not just on the penis itself. A condom doesn't cover all the spots where the virus can thrive. Using a condom helps, but it doesn't prevent it entirely. And having HPV puts you at higher risk for getting other STDs as well, which is the larger problem: The main way HPV can lead to infertility is that women who have it often also have undiagnosed gonorrhea, chlamydia or other STDs, and doctors won't automatically check. We know a woman who was diagnosed with HPV and then, six months later, found out she had AIDS—and had been infected with HIV for years without realizing it. Her gynecologist never suggested she get tested for other STDs after the HPV diagnosis. You have to be proactive and ask for testing if your doctor doesn't.

And again, HPV and its tagalong STDs can lead to PID, a serious danger to fertility.

Here are the two main ways that HPV treatment can contribute to infertility:

1. Some of the treatments for genital warts can harm your fertility. Warts may go away on their own, you may treat them with creams or gels, or a doctor may freeze them with liquid nitrogen, laser them off or electrocauterize them (heat them up with a metal probe to kill them). They should disappear within three months with treatment, though that's not a cure—it's really just for your comfort and to make it less likely for you to transmit the virus to others. HPV is contagious even when

warts aren't showing, but it's thought to be most contagious when you can see the warts.

2. If precancerous cells need to be removed, the surgery for removing them can lead to infertility. This can include cone biopsies (removing a piece of the cervix), LEEP (loop electro-surgical excision procedure—when a thin wire loop heated by electrical current is used to cut out abnormal tissue) or cryosurgery (freezing and destroying abnormal tissue).

In both cases, the treatments and surgeries can harm your fertility by weakening your cervix, interfering with cervical mucus production or creating scar tissue on your cervix and preventing sperm from reaching your egg.

If you go for an annual gynecological exam and your Pap smear comes back with abnormal results, it'll be reflexively tested for HPV because that can be a precursor to cervical cancer. Some people with HPV have normal Paps, however, so it's important to get tested.

There are now two vaccines approved in the United States to protect against HPV: Gardasil and Cervarix. They can prevent most cases of cervical cancer, vaginal and vulvar cancer, and genital warts, and the CDC recommends that girls and boys get vaccinated at age eleven or twelve before they become sexually active. Once someone has been exposed to HPV, the vaccines are less effective, but they still guard against types of the virus that you have not yet been exposed to. If you miss the earlier window, you can still get vaccinated up to age twenty-six. (It hasn't been studied enough in age groups beyond that to know if it's safe and effective at that point.) The vaccinations are given as a series of three injections in a six-month period because the immune system needs this much exposure to produce enough antibodies.

Note: If you've read that a researcher said the vaccine was danger-ous, this is not true. Neither is it true that any deaths have been linked to the vaccine. Diane Harper, a researcher who worked on the trials of the two vaccines, has made some critical comments about how the drugs are marketed because she doesn't want young women to believe they're invincible if they're vaccinated. She also questioned the long-term efficacy of the vaccines, since it's not known yet how long the protective effects last. But she also said in an article in *The Guardian,* "I fully support the HPV vaccines. I believe that in general, they are safe in most women."

# More about PID

We've told you that PID can cause infertility; now we'll tell you why. As the infection travels, it can get into your uterus, fallopian tubes, pelvis or ovaries. Once there, it causes inflammation, which can lead to scar tissue. Scar tissue can totally gum up the works because these organs are so small. Scars can block or twist your fallopian tubes, which are essential to getting you pregnant. Scarred fallopian tubes don't func-tion properly in helping the embryo reach the uterine cavity, where it implants and grows.

PID can also cause buildups of pus and fluids. If a fallopian tube and ovary get infected, you can get a tubo-ovarian abscess—a pus pocket that needs to be drained. It may be addressed with antibiot-ics, but, if not, then it can be drained using a large needle, or through a surgical procedure. Either way, it's really bad news: This kind of abscess causes infertility in more than 90 percent of cases.

You can also get a hydrosalpinx in either or both tubes. That's when an infection causes the tube to fill up with fluid and get very distended. It's not possible for the sperm to fertilize the egg when the tube is blocked like this. Hydrosalpinges are usually caused by STDs that have progressed to PID, but can also be caused by infection after abdominal surgery or abortion, endometriosis, tubal tuberculosis or intrauterine devices (IUDs).

If you have hydrosalpinges and you want to get pregnant, you have two options: surgical repair or IVF. Surgical repair is marginally successful at best and can lead to a tubal pregnancy. Reported success rates of surgically repaired hydrosalpinges are lower than IVF success rates. Even if you decide to go ahead with IVF, you are advised to have the infected tube or tubes removed first. Having untreated hydrosalpinges cuts your IVF success rate in half, despite the fact that IVF bypasses the fallopian tubes. Why? One theory is that fluids from the tubes may leak into the uterus, or possibly that the nutrition that should be going to the embryo is trapped in the tubes, but no one knows for sure. All they know is that if you're going to spend a lot of money for and invest a lot of your emotional capital in IVF treatments, you should improve your odds of success as much as possible and have those bloated tubes taken out. That brings the pregnancy rate back to normal, though there's still a slightly higher risk of miscarriage.

The symptoms of PID may be serious—usually involving pelvic pain and possibly nausea, vomiting, fever and unusual vaginal discharge—or they may be so mild that you don't even know anything is wrong. There are lots of women who have PID right now or have had it and don't realize it.

PID does get serious enough for hospitalization. Some infections are mild and clear up pretty easily with antibiotics (though any damage they've done to your reproductive organs is irreversible), while others are severe and life-threatening. Some women have lifelong pelvic pain because of all the scarring, even after an infection has been cured.

STDs are the main way a woman gets PID, but there are other ways, too: It can happen after an abortion or miscarriage, after insertion of an intrauterine insemination (IUI) device, after any kind of nonsterile gynecological surgery or procedure, from a ruptured appendix or from pelvic tuberculosis.

The CDC says that up to 15 percent of women who've had PID once become infertile, and that your odds of infertility increase with any subsequent infections.[2] If you've had PID three or more times, then your chance of infertility is over 70 percent. And the longer you go without treatment, the worse your odds are. Those who are symptomatic have worse fertility odds than those who didn't have any symptoms.

PID also significantly raises your risk of miscarriage and ectopic pregnancy. About 10 percent of pregnancies are ectopic after a woman has PID.

## Jamie Says . . .

A young woman came to my clinic for a second opinion after two failed IVF cycles at another clinic. She knew she had a hydrosalpinx that had come from untreated PID, but had elected not to remove it. I showed her the literature on the subject and told her that it was an unnecessary handicap; if she'd let me remove the infected tube before the next IVF cycle, it could double her chances of getting pregnant.

She agreed. I did the surgery, which was fairly simple, and then scheduled her next appointment for IVF. Then she called to tell me that she had missed her period.

"Well . . . do a pregnancy test," I said, and she humored me.

After two years of trying and two failed IVF cycles, she was pregnant. That's what can happen when you optimize the environment for pregnancy.

The same kind of thing occurred when I removed another patient's hydrosalpinx. She, too, had been to another clinic first and had several failed cycles where they had tried to implant two or three embryos at a time. After I did the surgery, I told her that her embryos looked good and I thought we should implant just one. Given her history, though, she wanted better odds than that—she asked me to implant two. I did. She has twins.

# Getting Tested

Unless you're showing obvious signs that a doctor can pick up on, you have to ask for STD testing. Don't count on your doctor telling you to get tested—few doctors will bring it up, for a bunch of reasons, not the least of which is that some patients get *offended* when they do.

## Kyra Says . . .

Oh, I was one of those offended patients.

While I was on assignment in Baghdad, shortly after my divorce, I kept getting bladder infections, so I went to see my doctor about it as soon as I got back.

"We'll have to test you for STDs," she said.

"What?!" I asked, all huffy. "I'm not sleeping around with any funky people. I can't even believe you're suggesting that."

I was dating by then, having sex with someone I'd met through mutual friends. It had been so long since I'd been in the dating

continued on page 30

world that I'd lost touch with the idea that you need to be seriously careful out there . . . and that indignant pride is for fools.

"I'm not trying to upset you. But people are not always honest, and any sexually active adults should be regularly tested, even couples," my doctor said. "Have you spoken with your partner about his history and testing?"

"Well, no."

I got over myself. When I saw the man I was dating again, I was ready with a flurry of questions. One cool thing about getting divorced was that it made me more gutsy. It affected me in lots of negative ways, but there were plenty of positive changes, too. After a short time, when I felt broken and worthless, I no longer cared to be obedient and placid; I grew a new kind of confidence and independence. I knew that I didn't need this new man if he couldn't show me respect by giving me straightforward answers. I had no time for drama—whether that was about love, sex, money or anything else. I realized I was worthy and didn't need to sacrifice myself anymore for someone else's comfort.

The older I got, the more pragmatic I got about sex—you probably don't know the whole history of the person you're sleeping with, even if you think you do. I was thankful to find out that I did not have any STDs. From that point on, I always made it a point to ask sexual questions of any guy I was dating—I wanted to know who he last had sex with (his ex-wife? a long-time girlfriend? just casual flings?), and not only whether he'd ever been tested for STDs, but when he had most recently been tested and what he'd been tested for. If I felt even the least bit uneasy with his answers, then I'd accompany him to the doctor so we could both be tested and feel comfortable knowing that we weren't going to pass anything to each other. Age provided me with the experience to know that not every relationship could or should be the "one," but that didn't mean I was going to live a sexless life until I found the guy I was (really) meant to marry.

You have absolutely nothing to lose by being candid and asking the pointed questions before getting into a sexual relationship with someone. A guy who isn't prepared to get tested for you and answer your questions is probably not someone you need in your life anyway.

And be aware that your annual Pap smear doesn't detect STIs or STDs. They can't be diagnosed that way, and your doctor won't test you without your consent, so you have to ask to be tested; your primary doctor or your OB/GYN can test you. Stay in control.

## If You Find Out You Have an STI

One common reaction women have to finding out they have an STI or STD is that they feel "dirty." But there's really nothing dirty about it—it's just bad luck. Anyone who has ever had any sexual contact with another human being can get an STI. It doesn't mean you're promiscuous. And, heck, even if you are— that doesn't make you a bad person, just a person who's had more sexual partners than average.

Your life and how you choose to live it is nobody's business, but you do have to be aware of the consequences of your choices and take precautions to protect yourself. Get tested regularly and have your partner tested.

# Which Ones Don't Mess with You

Common STDs that are unlikely to harm your fertility include tricho-monis (an infection caused by a parasite, which may cause unusual discharge), crabs (pubic lice), hepatitis B and HIV—though any kind of infection or disease can ultimately harm your fertility if it gets really bad or leads to secondary infections. For instance, if you have crabs and it causes intense itching, you may scratch enough to tear your vaginal tissue, which leaves it more susceptible to bacterial infection that could travel upward through your reproductive tract.

Herpes is not known to affect fertility, but if you have active lesions when you're about to give birth, then you may need a C-section to avoid transmitting it to your baby.

# STD Myths

## You Can't Have a Baby If You Have an Untreated STD

Not true. In some rare cases, you might not be able to have a vaginal delivery (if you have an active herpes outbreak, for instance), but the transmission of an STD to a baby is extremely rare and can usually be prevented by having a C-section, if necessary. Even if you're HIV-positive, you can still carry a baby as long as you take proper precautions. I'm not saying whether that's the right or wrong thing to do, but you can. You just can't breast-feed afterwards, because it carries the risk of transmitting HIV to the baby.

## You Can Get STDs from Toilet Seats

It's theoretically possible to get an STD from a toilet seat, but here's how it would have to happen: Since most germs can last only a very short time on a nonporous surface like a toilet seat, you'd have to use the restroom very quickly after the infected person did. You'd also have to either have a cut or sore on your butt or thighs and put that cut or sore right into contact with the spot where the infected person just sat, or you'd have to hump that toilet seat so severely that it comes into direct contact with your urethra or genital tract. Nor sure about you, but I rarely get that intimate with public toilets.

Most experts will tell you that it just doesn't happen. Period.

## If You Have Sex in the Water, You Won't Get an STD

Well, no. Even if you're swimming around in a chlorinated pool, the chlorine still won't kill an STD. Douching afterwards doesn't work, either.

## You Can't Get an STD from Oral Sex

Yes, you can. You totally can.

# How Not to Get an STD

Well, duh. Don't have sex.

What? Okay, fine, you're determined to have sex. Here are the ground rules:

1. **No CASUAL SEX.** Seriously, it's just not worth it. Some random guy in a bar is not going to give you such a mind-blowing orgasm that it's worth risking your life and risking the chance to have children in the future.

2. **USE CONDOMS ALWAYS.** Always, always, always. Listen, I hate to put it to you this way, but even if you're in a long-term relationship, you don't know if your guy is cheating on you. There have been scores of women who've found out the hard way because they got an STD and then realized that

their partner had to have picked it up recently. You also don't know if he has an STD from before your relationship and doesn't know it because it's asymptomatic. And don't just use a condom when you think the guy is going to ejaculate. There are fluids that come out before that point—called "pre-ejaculates"—that are just as prone to give you STDs. Use a condom or a dental dam when you're giving oral sex. Remember that you can get infected with many STDs through oral and anal sex, so don't think you can get away with using a condom only during intercourse.

3. **IF YOU'RE SHARING A SEX TOY, PUT A CONDOM ON IT.** Soap alone may not kill STIs, especially on porous materials like rubber. If the sex toy will be used by more than one person, put a fresh condom or dental dam on it on each time.

4. **MAKE NEW PARTNERS GET TESTED.** I know it can be a difficult thing to ask, but again, look what's at stake. You need to see the clean test results. It's not good enough to ask someone, "Hey, you don't have any STDs, right?" It's a fine start, but there's a high chance that he does and doesn't even know it, and there's also a chance that he knows it and wouldn't tell you. In one publicized case, a man named Phillipe Padieu intentionally infected dozens of women with HIV. Each of them thought that they were in an exclusive relationship with him, and at least one of his girlfriends asked him if he'd been tested for HIV. He said yes, and that he was clean. I'm sure you'd never intentionally date someone that schmucky, but still. You just never know. Get tested together for all the common STDs. Be there when he gets the results. If he passes, buy him some ice cream.

5. **Finish all treatments before having sexual contact
   again.** If either of you does find out you have a treatable STD,
   be sure you've finished treatment in full (don't just stop when
   you feel better or when you see the infection has cleared up)
   and you've had a follow-up test to make sure it's gone before
   you have sexual contact again. Otherwise, you're just setting
   yourself up for reinfection.

So be bold, be strong and go have yourself some great sex if that's
what you want to do . . . in the safest possible manner, of course. And
if you've already had problems with STDs, it's counterproductive to
spend time regretting things that can't be changed. If you find out that
it leads to problems with your fertility, that can often be fixed with
medications, minor surgery or both. And if not, there are still plenty of
other ways to have a baby aside from the "natural" way. Focus on the
options ahead of you instead of the mistakes behind you.

# Chapter 3
# Contraceptives and Abortions

You're onboard with this "I don't want an STD" thing and you're taking control of your body. Cool. Let's talk about your options.

## Different Types of Condoms

Latex condoms are the best method out there for STI and STD prevention. Period, full stop. Basically, everybody knows that...yet we still don't all use condoms all the time. That's why STIs are such a problem. We need to get you onboard with using one all the time. Every time, the whole time. The condom is your very best weapon in the fight to preserve your fertility.

One understandable reason why people don't want to use condoms is if they have latex allergies, which can make condom use pretty darn uncomfortable. You can get irritations, a rash, swelling, shortness of breath and, for an extra bit of fun, anaphylactic shock—which can actually kill you. Death by condom!

First, be sure that it's actually a latex allergy and not an allergy to the lubricant, spermicide or other chemicals used in a particular brand. I have a friend who thought she was allergic to condoms, when it turned out that it was just Trojans she couldn't handle. They made her all red and itchy. When she switched to Lifestyles, all was well.

But let's say you or your partner really are allergic to latex, which is most common among workers who are exposed to lots and lots of latex because they wear latex gloves, work with latex medical products, and so on. Your second-best option is to use polyurethane condoms (which are sold under some of the same major brands, and are labeled as such—like Trojan Supra Microsheer Polyurethane Condoms). Polyurethane condoms are just as effective at preventing STDs and pregnancy when they work properly, but they are slightly looser-fitting and less stretchy, making them a little more likely to break. Obviously, you lose the main benefit of the condom if it breaks, so your best bet is to stick with latex, if possible.

There are also lambskin condoms, but those are for preventing only pregnancy, not STDs. The lambskin (which is actually made of lamb intestines!) is porous—not porous enough for sperm to pass through, but porous enough for bacteria and viruses to get through.

One note: Don't use condoms with nonoxynol-9 (N9) on them! That's a spermicide. There's too little of it on condoms to be effective against pregnancy anyway, and the Food and Drug Administration (FDA) has been warning since 2007 that it can actually *increase* the chance of your getting HIV and other sexually transmitted infections. It works as a spermicide by damaging sperm cells' membranes, but it can also damage the cell lining of your vagina, rectum and cervix, making you more susceptible to STDs. How messed up is that?

Any products containing N9 now have to include a bunch of warnings on their labels, including this: "Studies have raised safety concerns that products containing the spermicide nonoxynol-9 can irritate the vagina and rectum. Sometimes this irritation has no symptoms. This irritation may increase the risk of getting HIV/AIDS from an infected partner." So why do condom makers keep making condoms with this ineffective and potentially harmful spermicide? Because people don't read warning labels. They see *spermicide* and they think, *Extra protection. Cool.* But not you. You're wise. You read stuff.

## Why Do Condoms Fail?

When condoms are used the right way, just one in one hundred women will get pregnant in a year. But when they're not used right, fifteen women in one hundred will.

If you want your condom to actually do its job, it can't break. Here are the major causes of condom breakage or failure:

- **NOT ENOUGH LUBRICATION:** If you're not quite...there... then use a condom-safe lubricant. You can't just use any old thing, like Vaseline or baby oil—those can weaken the condom. Use a water- or silicone-based lubricant that specifies it's compatible with latex (or polyurethane) condoms. Oil-based lubes are trouble.

- **NOT APPLIED PROPERLY:** You have to pinch the tip while you're rolling it on to prevent air bubbles. Leave some room at the tip for the good stuff. Also, unroll it just a tiny bit first to make sure you're not trying to put it on inside out. If you start to put it on the wrong way, and then you turn it the right way, you've already potentially gotten pre-ejaculate and bacteria or viruses on the side that's now about to be inside one of your orifices. Save your orifices! Toss it out and get a new condom!

- **EXPIRED:** Old condoms dry out and get brittle, making them more prone to breaking. There's an expiration date printed on every individual condom package. Take a quick peek before tearing it open (which, by the way, should be done with your hands and not anything sharp and pointy).

- **INCORRECTLY STORED:** You can't leave a condom wrapper open and use it later. It'll dry out. You also can't leave it in a hot place, like on a windowsill or in a car's glove compartment in the summer. Before you open a condom package, squish the condom around in there to make sure you can still feel an air bubble.

- **NOT TAKEN OFF PROPERLY:** Don't wait too long after sex to take off the condom. If you wait until a guy is getting soft, the condom can easily slip off or get loose, and then both his penis and his semen can go rogue on you. Instead, soon after he ejaculates, he or you should hold the condom at the base of the penis and have him pull out and take it off. Don't keep going after he ejaculates, even if he doesn't get soft right away. The condom can still fall off because now it's all slippery inside. Always use a new second condom if you're going for round 2.

- **WRONG FIT:** Most guys fit into regular-size condoms. However, guys who are larger or thicker than average should buy large (or extra-large) condoms, and guys who are smaller should buy snug-fit condoms. Notice they don't say *small*, because that would just be mean. Instead they say things like, "For those men who want a snugger fit." If you're not sure what's appropriate for your guy, there's a size chart at www.condomania.com. Click "Condoms by size."

# Condoms and Students

Society is still a little squeamish about handing out condoms in public places. The American Academy of Pediatrics has openly recommended that condoms should be freely distributed in high schools, particularly in communities where STI/STD rates are high. They note that adolescents get 25 percent of all STDs, and that's mostly because they don't use condoms consistently. And some high schools do follow this advice—they make condoms available in the nurse's office or a health resource room—but many others, particularly in religious communities, don't.

Parents in religious communities have freaked out when condoms have been made available to their teens. They think it will encourage their kids to have sex, when the truth is that there's no proof of that—it doesn't seem that kids have sex any earlier when condoms are freely available, just that they'll actually use condoms more often when they do have sex. The same applies to sex education classes—some states teach students about contraceptives, whereas others don't. Texas, Arkansas and Arizona don't mandate sex ed, but if schools choose to teach it, they must stress abstinence only . . . and those states have some of the highest rates of teen pregnancy in the country.

Some states, such as New York, have mandated condom availability in schools. New York City schools are required to have a health resource room with condoms available at least ten periods a week. However—and here's a bit of a complicated issue—parents can opt out from their kids receiving condoms. So a staff member has to check the student's ID number to make sure that his or her parent hasn't disallowed the student from receiving condoms. That still creates a barrier for all students, because it means that a student has to show his or her face to a staff member and ask for condoms and get approval. Such a big part of the reason teens don't consistently use condoms is because they're embarrassed to go buy them—they don't want people to know that they're having sex. Having to check in with a school staff member is going to be a deterrent for a lot of these students.

Even on the college level, and even in major cities, there is strong resistance to making condoms freely available. At Boston College, a small group of students began handing out condoms along with literature about STDs in specially designated dorm rooms and on the street on certain days, and the college ordered them to stop in 2013, with the dean of students and director of student life signing a letter that said, in part, "The distribution of condoms is not congruent with our values and traditions" and threatening the group with disciplinary action if they continued. The college has a page about sexually transmitted infections on its website, and the only suggestion it makes for avoiding them is abstinence.

Creating shame and barriers like this helps STDs flourish and makes people feel bad about their bodies. It also creates problems for people's overall health and future fertility. Meanwhile, a few miles over at Boston University, a seminar about sexual pleasure and contraceptives has been part of freshmen orientation, and free condoms are readily available in the student health center—so it is school-specific.

You might think that the problem is that we're tight-lipped about sex in the United States and that counties known for being more open about sexuality would be more apt to distribute condoms in schools but, for the most part, that's not the case. Just as in the United States, there are some schools around the world that distribute free condoms, and some that don't; some that require parental permission and some that don't. In one part of the UK, for instance, they offer a little key fob—like the plastic loyalty cards you might keep on your keychain for your favorite grocery or drugstore—called a "C Card" to people under the age of twenty. To get one, you have to speak to a school nurse or youth professional about sex and contraception, or answer a questionnaire online and print it out and bring it to a place that distributes these cards. Then you can use that card to get free condoms at more than seventy locations, meaning that you don't have to ask again. You just swipe your card.

## Kyra Says . . .

When I went to Antarctica to film a documentary, one of the funniest things I noticed right away was that there were buckets of free condoms in every public bathroom I visited.

It seemed really odd until I learned about the logistics of the situation; you're at the mercy of the weather gods there, and you can't just come and go as you please. Taking a plane to or from Antarctica is an exercise in patience because your departure and arrival times can change frequently if the weather doesn't cooperate.

So imagine being pregnant in Antarctica. It's not as if you can just hop in the car and take a leisurely drive to the hospital whenever you feel like it, and your health has to be a major priority because of the lack of access to doctors and clinics. There are three American research bases in Antarctica where scientists work in extremely rough conditions and don't have a whole lot to do when they're not working . . . which can lead to boredom sex. Lots of people are shacking up.

It's under these conditions that massive numbers of condoms are shipped to the continent—one report said that in 2008, a base of 125 scientists got a shipment of 16,500 condoms. That's why there are condoms *everywhere*. It became a running joke between my coworkers. My producer thought it was hilarious to stick condoms in the oddest places—when I went to do an interview, I'd open my backpack and a dozen condoms would spill out. So I got her back and stuck condoms in her boots. This went back and forth the whole time we were there, but she got the last laugh because she mailed a letter from Antarctica to my home address, and when I arrived back home, I found a condom in the envelope.

This is possible because there are no kids or teens around these research bases, so there's no issue of parents complaining that condoms are too freely available.

Now what happens if you're in a long-term committed relationship and you decide you can forgo condoms, despite our stellar advice, or you just want a backup method of birth control in addition to condoms? Here are your other picks and how they can affect your fertility.

# Birth Control Pills

Birth control pills can have a number of side effects, but messing up your fertility is not one of them. In fact, it's just the opposite—being on birth control pills for years can make it easier for you to conceive afterwards! I know...you'd expect the opposite, right?

The exact reason is not certain, but this is what we know: Most of the time, even if you've been on the pill for years and years, your fertility will return to normal within three months after you stop taking it. Now here's the cooler part: Researchers from Brunel University in the UK surveyed nearly nine thousand pregnant women and found that the longer a woman had been taking the pill, the more likely it was for her to get pregnant within six months off the pill. So not only did it not harm a woman's chances of getting pregnant but, on average, she got pregnant faster than women who didn't take the pill at all or who'd taken it for a shorter time.

The pill contains two forms of synthetic hormones that work to prevent ovulation. Once you stop taking the pill, those hormones leave your body quickly—that's why it's so important to remember to take the pill close to the same time every day to keep the hormone levels up. Skipping even one day could lead to a pregnancy. That's one reason why the pill can be a good choice if you're considering trying to get pregnant fairly soon, or if you're at least open to the possibility.

## The Patch and the Implant

Ortho-Evra is a contraceptive skin patch. You put on a new one once a week for three weeks, then skip the fourth week and get your period.

The implant (Implanon or Nexplanon) is even easier: A doctor implants a rod the size of a match under the skin of your upper arm, and it prevents pregnancy for up to three years. When you want to get pregnant, you just have it removed.

Pregnancy rates are about the same for both of these; your fertility returns to normal quickly and you can get pregnant just as easily as a woman who's never taken any kind of birth control.

## Depo-Provera

Depo-Provera is a shot you get in your arm or butt that contains synthetic progesterone. It's a lot more convenient than the pill because you don't have to remember to take it every day—you just go to the doctor once every twelve weeks for a shot. However, it doesn't leave your system as easily as the pill does.

Regardless of how long you've been on Depo-Provera, it can take much longer for you to conceive afterwards. It's not a common side effect, but it does happen. If you think there's any chance you might want to get pregnant in the next year, then this is not the birth control you want to use.

## IUDs

Intrauterine devices (IUDs) are flexible T-shaped plastic devices that a doctor inserts into your uterus to prevent pregnancy. There are two tyes: hormonal and copper. The hormonal IUD releases a form of progestin and can prevent pregnancy for three to five years, and the copper IUD releases copper into the uterus, creating an environment that's toxic to sperm. It can last up to twelve years.

There was a time in the 1970s when IUDs were very dangerous, but today's IUDs are much safer.

The main risk is uterine perforation, which is very rare (about one in one thousand), and there is a very slight risk that you can't carry a baby after your uterus has been perforated. But take that statistic however you like; it's an extremely effective birth control method (99 percent success rate) that also has high user satisfaction ratings. It seems that uterus perforation usually occurs at the time the device is inserted, and it can be repaired. So if you're going to get an IUD, make sure the person who inserts it is experienced and reputable. You don't want some quack poking holes in your womb.

## Abortions and the Morning-After Pill

Now let's get into a stickier topic: abortion. Nearly half of all pregnancies in the United States are unplanned and 22 percent of all pregnancies end in abortion—a statistic that bears out in the fertility clinic. Jamie says that about 25–30 percent of the women who come to him for infertility treatment have terminated a pregnancy in the past. Will having an abortion affect your future fertility? He says most likely not. Abortion generally does not cause a problem unless the patient gets an infection afterwards that could damage the tubes or the uterine lining, or the lining is perforated during the procedure, both of which are rare.

Taking antibiotics before and after an abortion can stave off an infection, and if you do get one, treating it quickly can save your fertility.

There are two types of abortions: medical and surgical. A medical abortion is where you take the drug mifepristone (formerly called RU486) or misoprostol to block progesterone and end a pregnancy that's less than forty-nine days along. If you're more than forty-nine days along, your only option is a surgical abortion, where a practitioner uses either a vacuum to suction out the uterus or a dilation and curettage (D&C) procedure where the practitioner dilates the cervix and then uses surgical instruments to scrape out the uterus.

There is obviously a greater chance of infection and complications with surgical abortions, as opposed to medical abortions (which are noninvasive). And the further along the pregnancy is, the greater the chance for complications. About 2.5 in 100 women will have some kind of complication following a medical abortion, and about 4 in 100 following a surgical abortion, but few of those complications result in infertility. The ones that do threaten future fertility are things such as damage to the cervix, perforation of the uterus from a surgical device or the development of PID if a woman develops an infection after surgery.

There is also a slightly increased risk of miscarriage in any subsequent pregnancy after an abortion. The reason is unknown.

Jamie says that he sees a lot of women at the fertility clinic who now feel guilty because they think they're being punished for having an abortion earlier in their lives. "They forget the struggle they went through to make what was probably one of the hardest decisions in their lives," he says. "They came up with that as the right decision at the time because, most likely, it was the right decision. If they had a video now and could see the situation they were in at the time, they would remember why they did it. Infertility brings up feelings of pain, and pain has no integrity. How do women manage their pain? Sometimes by stirring up old pain and attaching it to the new situation and getting stuck. It's not helpful to punish yourself afterwards."

The "would'ves" and "could'ves" are not a good place to remain, and it's not your doctor's place to judge you. It's up to you to make the best choices you can for each situation and time of your life.

The morning-after pill (there are different brands—some available over the counter at drugstores, and one by prescription) is a drug you can take up to five days after having sex. It just prevents your body from ovulating for longer than usual so that there's no egg for the sperm to meet, and it has no lasting effect on your fertility, even if it's taken frequently.

## Bottom Line

If you want to perfectly preserve your fertility, the best way is to have no sex life at all...but how practical (or fun) is that? Just do the best you can. Arm yourself with knowledge about how to properly use condoms (and, hey, there are YouTube videos on this stuff if you need a little more instruction—no shame needed! Seriously, you can practice on a banana or a dildo or whatever you have on hand that's vaguely penis-shaped if you're worried about coming across awkwardly with your partner). Promise yourself that you'll speak up if something goes wrong—like if you see your partner try to reuse a condom he accidentally started putting on inside out. I know it can be difficult to "correct" your partner or tell him to do something that he isn't doing on his own. But this is your vagina and your life we're talking about. If you find out one day that you can't have a baby because of that one time you let your boyfriend get away with not putting on a second condom after the first one broke, you're going to be mad. Trust us. Or don't. But we're still right!

# Chapter 4
# Lifestyle Differences for Fertility

You probably know that there are certain things you'll have to stop doing once you get pregnant—obvious stuff like smoking and drinking. But the same sorts of things can also affect your fertility before you stop.

## Smoking and Secondhand Smoke

As if anyone needs another reason to quit smoking, besides the whole "There's a fair shot you're going to die a slow and agonizing death from it," smoking is the same as feeding your eggs poison.

The American Society for Reproductive Medicine also recognizes that people don't know how much smoking may harm fertility. They did a survey and found that 99 percent of people knew that smoking could cause lung cancer and respiratory disease and 96 percent knew it could cause heart disease, but only 22 percent said they knew it could cause infertility, and only 17 percent knew it caused early menopause. The organization published a fact sheet that explains a few simple truths[1]:

1. Prevalence of infertility is higher in smokers than nonsmokers.

2. It takes smokers longer to conceive than nonsmokers, both naturally and through IVF. It requires twice as many IVF cycles, on average, for smokers. And do you know how expensive those IVF cycles are? When trying to conceive naturally, 54 percent more smokers than nonsmokers don't conceive for more than a year.

3. Active smoking by either partner causes infertility problems, and inhaling secondhand smoke regularly is nearly as damaging as if you were the one smoking.

4. Cigarette smoke harms a woman's ovaries. How much harm depends in part on how long and how much you smoked.

5. Smoking can speed up menopause by one to four years, depending on how long and how much you smoked. It kills off your eggs at a faster rate than normal, so you lose your fertility sooner.

6. Cigarette smoke can interfere with the ability of the cells in your ovaries to make estrogen, which results in more genetic abnormalities.

Remember, all of this is true even if you quit smoking before you try to get pregnant. If you do smoke while you're pregnant (and how in the world could you even think of doing that?), you're significantly increasing your risk of miscarriage, and the baby's chance of sudden infant death syndrome (SIDS), along with all the other problems we've already discussed.

It's so important for both partners to quit—quit now. If you live with a smoker, get him or her to quit or move out, or move out yourself. You can't afford to deal with the effects of secondhand smoke.

Short-term fertility does generally return to normal within a few months of quitting, but the eggs that have been killed off or damaged are done for. So don't fool yourself into thinking that it's okay to wait until you're actually pregnant; now is the time to quit if you're concerned about making your fertility last.

Jamie says that when he sees older women at his clinic who have been smokers, their ovarian reserves are usually lower than average. There's no way to pinpoint if that's a direct result of smoking or if that's combined with other factors or just plain bad luck, but he says that it's common sense that the various chemicals in cigarette and cigar smoke are no good for your reproductive organs. "If you put something toxic in your body, you're not going to make a biologically functioning system work better." You can get some recovery from quitting, but you never return to where you would have been if you'd never started. It becomes just one more hurdle on your fertility journey, and that hurdle gets higher the longer you smoke.

## Kyra Says . . .

I always knew that I couldn't and wouldn't smoke during pregnancy—the dangers of that are pretty well-known now. You risk having a low-birth-weight baby, and/or a preemie with all sorts of complications, so I knew I was going to have to give up my beloved cigarettes when I started trying to conceive. My girlfriend Leanne waited until the last second and flushed her last cigarette when she got her positive pregnancy test.

But neither of us realized that we could be harming our odds of conceiving in the first place, or raising the risk of birth defects even if we quit as soon as we got pregnant.

## Quitting Smoking

If you're already pregnant or trying to conceive, then it's best to go cold turkey or quickly wean yourself off cigarettes if you can, rather than using nicotine replacement therapies. But assuming you're not at that stage yet, nicotine replacements such as the patch or gum are a lot safer than continuing to smoke—so use them if it helps. Pick a quit date not too far into the future and plan for the cravings that will almost certainly arise. Keep yourself busy that first week and make sure you have substitutes ready for your oral cravings, like gum, lollipops and mints. And drink plenty of water and juice.

Here are some other resources that many people say have helped them:

- **www.quitnet.com:** A community where everyone is trying to, or has, quit smoking. It's a place to check in, stay accountable, get support and trade tips.
- *Alan Carr's Easy Way to Quit Smoking* by **Alan Carr** (duh): This is a book that can change the way you think about why you smoke.
- **Bupropion** (brand name Zyban): This is a prescription antidepressant medication that can help with cravings. You start taking it a week before your quit date and continue taking it for seven to twelve weeks.
- **Hypnosis:** You can go for individual or group hypnosis sessions to help train your brain to be grossed out by cigarettes.

# Caffeine

The studies about caffeine's effects on fertility aren't conclusive. Some studies say that caffeine intake can harm fertility, other studies show no effect, and one study even showed improved pregnancy rates among people who drank caffeinated drinks. Do what you want with that information. Common sense tells us that it's a stimulant that's known to have harmful effects on other systems of the body, so there's a chance that it could also have harmful effects on your fertility or reproductive organs, even if the studies are not yet clear.

Once you are actively trying to conceive, then it's definitely time to cut back on caffeine if you have a strong habit. Be aware that you may have to wean yourself down from caffeine. It's an addictive substance, and if you go from several cups of coffee or cola a day to none, you could get headaches, suffer from anxiety and feel irritable. Gradually reduce your consumption over a few weeks.

## Jamie Says . . .

I advise my infertility patients to have no more than two cups of coffee or its equivalent per day (don't forget that there's caffeine in chocolate, tea, many carbonated drinks, energy drinks and some medications like those for migraine relief). As with many other things, the key is moderation. A moderate amount of caffeine during pregnancy has never been shown to harm a fetus, whereas excessive amounts (more than two cups of coffee per day) can be harmful, leading to an increase in miscarriages and low-birth-weight babies.

# Alcohol

There have been several studies trying to determine how alcohol affects fertility, and the consensus is that drinking excessively does screw up your fertility. It's dehydrating, which is detrimental to babymaking, and binge drinking poisons your body in all sorts of ways, including messing up your hormone levels (too much estrogen, not enough progesterone). It hinders women's ovulation and reduces men's sperm parameters: counts, motility and morphology. Moderate to high levels of drinking are also associated with endometriosis. The question becomes where to draw the line—how much drinking is too much? One study determined that "too much" was just four drinks a week.

This study of more than 2,500 couples in the Boston area undergoing fertility treatments showed that the women who reported that they drank at least four alcoholic beverages a week had 16 percent lower odds of an IVF cycle resulting in a live birth than women who drank less. When both partners in a couple drank at least four alcoholic beverages a week, the odds were even worse: 21 percent lower birth rates than couples who drank less.

It's possible that alcohol affects couples who are already infertile differently from how it affects fertile couples, because other studies have not shown the same kind of effect from moderate drinking.

One of the biggest concerns women have about trying to conceive is if it's okay to go out for drinks during that period. Jamie again suggests moderation—he tells his infertility patients that if they want to have a couple of drinks a week (but not overdo it), that's fine. Light drinking is not known to have an effect on fertility—there have been conflicting studies, with at least two suggesting that light wine consumption actually *promotes* fertility (lowering the amount of time to conception), but nothing convincing to show it has a detrimental effect if you have just two or three drinks a week.

## Kyra Says . . .

I chose to completely cut out alcohol during the fertility process, and didn't have even a sip during my pregnancy. In my opinion and experience, why even take the risk? If you're trying so hard to have a baby, how does it make sense to do anything that could harm your chances or negatively affect that beautiful child growing inside you?

# Recreational Drugs

Recreational drugs as a category have less of an effect on a woman's fertility than you might think. If taken while you're pregnant, drugs have major effects on a fetus's development in the womb, but most drugs don't have long-term effects on your fertility beforehand. In the case of most recreational drugs, the effect is much worse on men's sperm than it is on women's reproductive systems.

Marijuana is not known for having a major effect on women's fertility, but heavy use can disrupt your menstrual cycle. It does lower sperm count and testosterone in men. Heroin and cocaine are both associated with ovulatory dysfunction, and steroids can cause you not to ovulate at all. These effects are relatively reversible by stopping.

If you've done LSD, you may have heard the rumor that it causes chromosomal damage—that's been roundly debunked. The only time LSD affects your fertility or adds to the possibility of birth defects is while you're actively using it. As long as you stop using it prior to trying to conceive, it shouldn't be a problem.

Nitrous oxide (laughing gas) is another drug that has a proven connection to infertility: After animal studies showed that female rats exposed to about the same levels of nitrous oxide that you'd find in a dental office were less fertile than those that hadn't been exposed, researchers tested their results on dental assistants next. They found that dental assistants who were exposed to high levels of nitrous oxide (at least five hours a week of exposure—not that they were inhaling the stuff directly themselves, but just that they were in the room when patients were breathing it) were only 41 percent as likely to get pregnant each cycle than women who weren't exposed to the drug. Be careful about using this as a "party drug" if you want to preserve your fertility.

It takes about ninety days for an egg to mature, so—assuming there's been no permanent damage—that's the minimum amount of time you need to be drug-free before getting pregnant if you want the best odds of having a healthy baby.

# Exercise

Exercise is a great thing. Never let it be said that Kyra Phillips or Jamie Grifo are discouraging exercise. But there does come a point when it can actually cause you to stop ovulating.

We'll get into this in greater depth in the section about BMI (chapter 9), but, in short, competitive athletes—and distance runners in particular—often stop menstruating altogether. If you exercise a lot and your periods are irregular, then you'll want to cut back before you start trying to conceive.

A woman named Kristine Fretwell was a competitive bodybuilder until she realized that although it was making the outside of her body look terrific, it was severely screwing up her insides. She stopped getting her period in her third month of training for her first competition, which she thought was just a sign that her training was paying off—she knew it meant that her body fat was dropping very low. However, it led to infertility for two years, even after she stopped competing.

"Just for the record, it took me literally two weeks to get pregnant with my daughter, so we never figured the second one would be a problem," she wrote on her blog.

She did eventually get pregnant and had another daughter, but it took quite a while for her menstrual cycles to straighten out to allow her to conceive again, and she says that if she had known then the effects of intensive training, she wouldn't have competed.

But in addition to women like Kristine, a surprising recent study out of Denmark showed that even among women who aren't competitive athletes, doing what the researchers classified as "vigorous" exercise (running, fast cycling, aerobics, gymnastics and swimming) at least five hours a week was associated with longer times to conceive among women who were not obese. It didn't have any negative effect on obese women, but women with healthy BMIs took longer to get pregnant the more vigorous exercise they did each week. On the other hand, women who said they did what the researchers classified as "moderate" exercise (brisk walking, leisurely cycling, gardening and golfing) for more than five hours a week got pregnant at slightly better than average rates—they were 18 percent more likely to conceive each cycle as compared to women who did little to no exercise.[2]

Showing that there's an association doesn't mean it's cause and effect, however. There could be other factors that caused the "vigorous exercisers" to take longer to get pregnant, but you might still want to take that into consideration and switch to more moderate exercise when you're ready to start trying for a baby. The researchers from that study recommend thirty minutes a day of moderate exercise, walking in particular, because it keeps your whole body in tune better—and that includes better pregnancies with less pain and shorter labors. So get off your butt and start walking.

# Douching

Quit yer douching. Seriously, it does more harm than good, even if you're not trying to conceive. Your glorious vagina is made to be a self-cleaning mechanism, and it doesn't need you shoving vinegar and chemicals up there to help it along.

In every vagina, there are good and bad bacteria, and you need a balance or there can be problems. If you have a yeast infection, for instance, then you have too many bad bacteria in there, and probiotics—as in yogurt—help you add good bacteria to restore the balance.

When you douche, you're washing away not only the bad bacteria but the good as well. You're screwing up your vagina's whole routine. It's like Rainman in there—it doesn't want its routine disrupted. It wants to watch Wapner and drive slow in the driveway.

In addition, if you do have an infection—which might be why you're douching in the first place (likely to get rid of odor or a weird discharge), then douching can push the infection higher up into your uterus, fallopian tubes and ovaries. You know that's trouble.

Douching puts you at higher risk for vaginal infections and STDs and can lead to permanent damage to your reproductive tract.

Even happy, healthy vaginas can have a little odor to them, and they're not meant to be the driest, neatest little organs. If you're douching because you don't feel "clean," there might be something else wrong—are you itchy or uncomfortable, or is there a foul odor, or do you have a strange discharge or stuff like that? Then skip the douche and just go to your doctor. There's nothing to be embarrassed about. It could be an infection that needs to be treated, and once it's treated, you won't even have to think about douching anymore. Your vagina's good. Worry about other stuff, like how giant pandas are in danger of extinction. Man, those things are cute.

# Rethink Your Period Products

Vaginas are ultra-absorbent. Medications or chemicals quickly get into the bloodstream when inserted in the vagina, which is why you have to be extra-careful about what you're doing "down there." A new study by Women's Voices for the Earth brought up a disturbing truth about feminine care products: For all practical purposes, their ingredients are unregulated.[3]

Products such as feminine sprays and powders are considered cosmetics, and while the law states that they have to be free of poisonous substances that might harm people who use them normally, it's a self-regulating industry: They're not required to do any testing or submit safety information to the FDA. You can imagine how well the honor system works.

Tampons and pads are classified as medical devices, and the law says that means their manufacturers don't need to disclose their ingredients. The study authors were particularly concerned about tampons, because those are inserted into the permeable vaginal tissue for hours at a time for several days a month, which is a lot of exposure.

When they reviewed the scientific literature, here's what they found:

- **DIOXINS AND FURANS:** A 2002 study found dioxins and furans in all four brands of tampons tested. Dioxins and furans are toxic substances that are by-products of manufacturing processes. In the case of tampons, they're likely by-products of the chlorine bleaching most tampons

go through before they're boxed up and sold to you—
because customers associate the color white with cleanliness
and purity. The EPA notes that, in animal studies, animals
exposed to these toxins experienced changes in their hormone
levels, impaired fertility, decreased immune functions and
harm to their fetuses; human studies have shown changes
in hormone levels. You obviously don't want to mess with
your hormones, particularly when fertility is a concern.

- **PESTICIDES:** A 2013 study found eight pesticides in
  a popular brand of tampons, two of which are classified as
  "probable carcinogens" by the EPA. Most tampons are made
  of cotton and/or synthetics, such as rayon and viscose,
  and cotton is one of the most pesticide-laden crops
  in existence.

- **FRAGRANCE:** The word *fragrance* on any cosmetic or health
  product label is maddening because it can mean almost
  anything. By calling something a "fragrance," manufacturers
  get away with not having to disclose any of hundreds of
  chemicals that may be in their products. Some of those
  chemicals are harmless; some aren't. You have no way of
  knowing from the label. But nothing with a "fragrance"
  belongs in or next to your vagina anyway. In addition to
  the possible carcinogens and reproductive- and hormone-
  affecting chemicals that may be present, there's also the simple
  fact that many fragrances are irritating to vulnerable vaginal
  and vulvar tissue, causing problems with rashes and infections.
  And, as you know, any infection—if it gets bad enough—can
  travel into your reproductive system and harm your fertility.
  There's just no reason to risk it.

You probably have also heard that tampons increase your risk of toxic shock syndrome (TSS), which is generally a problem if tampons are left in too long. You should change your tampon every four to six hours (and definitely not leave it in more than eight hours), using the lowest absorbency that works, to minimize your risks. TSS is a very serious and sometimes deadly problem; however, it does not affect your fertility, so if you've had it, there's one worry you can cross off your list. In studies, it hasn't been shown to hinder pregnancy or cause birth defects.

## Better Feminine Care Options

Moms have used popular brand tampons and sanitary pads for a long time and most of us have not ended up with fertility problems as a result; of course you can continue to use your preferred product and know that you'll probably be okay. But if you want to be as safe as possible, then look for organic, chlorine-free tampons and sanitary pads. They may not be on every grocery or drugstore shelf, but they're out there. Natracare, Seventh Generation and Dr. Mercola have their own brands, which you can find online.

You may also want to try a menstrual cup. They're soft silicone (or other nonlatex material) cups that you insert into your vagina and empty regularly, and they come in various sizes and shapes. Most are reusable; some are disposable. If you're not grossed out by the idea, there are a number of benefits (environmental, economic and health). They can be safely used longer than tampons (up to twelve hours without changing), but also there's the caveat that you must follow the cleaning instructions very carefully or risk getting an infection. There's sort of an underground cult movement feel to the menstrual cup aficionados—if you search online, you can find scores of women singing the praises of their favorite brands (some of the more popular ones are DivaCup, Moon Cup, Softcup, The Keeper and Instead).

# Antibacterial Everything

There are two main active ingredients in antibacterial stuff: triclosan or alcohol.

Triclosan is a chemical that's been used since the 1960s in hospital settings to prevent infections, but only in about the last decade has it become ever-present in our consumer lives—especially in hand soap, body wash, shampoo, mouthwash, alcohol-free hand sanitizers and toothpaste. Most of us now have a detectible level present in our bodies, and it's actually getting harder to find hand soaps that are not antibacterial. About 75 percent of all the hand soaps on the market now are antibacterial.

There is controversy about whether or not the overuse of antibacterial products will lead to bacterial resistance—when bacteria mutate and become stronger and antibiotics are no longer effective. Some scientists say yes, but the majority say no. That debate is beyond the scope of this book, but one thing we can mention is that triclosan is known to be an endocrine disruptor in animals, which means that it could affect your fertility if those effects also occur in humans, and the FDA doesn't believe it offers any benefit over regular soap-and-water hand washing. The chemical is under FDA review right now to determine if it poses any threats to human health, and if it has any real benefits. We'd file it under "avoid when possible." Regular soap and water should be the main staple in your house.

Most hand sanitizing gels and foams, however, work by using alcohol to kill germs. A sanitizer with at least 60 percent alcohol is very effective and helpful for preventing bacterial infection and somewhat effective at preventing viruses. Bacteria do not build up resistance to alcohol. You can feel safe using alcohol-based hand sanitizers without worrying about your fertility. The best germ prevention is still washing your hands with soap and water for at least twenty seconds (the length of time it takes to sing "Happy Birthday" twice, slowly), but when that's not possible, hand sanitizers are your second-best option.

# Get Your Annual Exams

Of course you know that you're supposed to have an OB/GYN check-up every year. Do you do it? If you're one of those women who puts it off, don't. It's your first line of defense for finding out of there's anything going wrong that you need to fix. You need to get those annual Paps and exams to check for cancer, STIs and infections, as well as to make sure there's nothing else wonky going on with your reproductive system. If you have trouble remembering, then tie it to an important event, like your birthday. Agree to schedule your annual visit within a week of your birthday each year.

If you want to know where you stand with fertility issues before you're ready to start trying, it's a good idea to have your regular OB/GYN do an ovarian reserve test—a simple blood test to determine approximately how many eggs you have left in your stash. What they're checking for is called "diminished ovarian reserve," or "not enough eggs." They score you against other women your age to determine where you stack up. Some women at thirty already have diminished ovarian reserves and are headed for early menopause, whereas others still have solid ovarian reserves at forty. And you can't tell who's who by looking at them.

Why do gynecologists not talk to you about this simple test at your annual exam? I DON'T KNOW. But they should. Because why wouldn't you want to know as early as possible if there's a potential problem?

Well, I'll rephrase that. It's possible you wouldn't want to know because it adds more pressure. Say you *are* that thirty-year-old with diminished ovarian reserves, and you're not in a steady relationship and your job is not all that secure. What do you do with that information? Do you freak out and vow to marry the next guy who wolf-whistles at you at a construction site? Do you sell a kidney so you can freeze your eggs? It's opening Pandora's box, and you may not be prepared for the answer you get. But if you *want* to be informed and you're ready to hear whatever may come, then you most likely need to ask for it rather than wait for the doctor to mention it to you. Gynecologists can be squeamish about bringing up fertility stuff because they don't want to offend or scare away patients. They don't know what's going on in your mind unless you volunteer it, and women have been known to leave their gynecologists for perceived insensitivity or "prying" into their personal lives by asking about fertility issues. And they get screwed both ways . . .

"My stupid OB/GYN told me that if I want to have a baby, I should hurry up. I'm only thirty-eight! What a jerk!"

"Why didn't my OB/GYN warn me that my fertility was in decline? He never warned me and now I'm thirty-eight and infertile!"

See? So they basically wait for you to bring it up. So go ahead and ask, and insurance will likely cover the test. The downside is that the test the OB/GYN does will probably just measure your follicle-stimulating hormone (FSH) level, which is a good test but not as comprehensive as what a reproductive endocrinologist would do. What happens with this test is that on day 3 of your menstrual cycle (day 1 is the first day of your period—not spotting, but the full-on week o' fun), he'll do a blood test to see how much of this hormone you have in your system. FSH is one of the most important hormones in pregnancy. As you age, your FSH score gets higher early in your cycle because the hormones are working harder to stimulate your tired old ovaries to make good follicles. When you go into menopause, your FSH score stays high forever because your body is still trying to get you pregnant even though you don't have any eggs left. Kind of sad, really. It's like a guy sitting around waiting for years for his girlfriend to come back, even though she married a pilot named Gustavus and moved to Tahiti and forgot her ex's name.

So anyway, as a rough guideline, you want your FSH level to be under 15 mIU/ml—under 10 is better—but the thresholds vary from lab to lab. What's high in one lab may be normal in another. It's important for you to know what's normal in your lab.

FSH levels may vary from month to month and may be affected by factors such as stress and illness, so one high FSH score isn't the end of the world. But it does give you a starting point for understanding what's going on in your babymaking factory.

# Final Thoughts

We believe that knowledge is power, and that women who learn all they can make good decisions. We hope you've learned a little more about how the everyday decisions you make can affect your fertility, and that you won't beat yourself up if you haven't done everything "perfectly" up to now. Nobody does it all perfectly, and most women get pregnant despite that. But now you know a few more ways to protect your body and your eggs.

When Jamie counsels his patients who ask about things like whether or not they *really* need to quit drinking or smoking when trying to conceive, he tells them to think about the worst possible outcome of that decision and then figure out if they can live with it. Either way, they have their answer.

# Chapter 5

# Medications and Health Conditions That Can Affect Your Fertility

There are lots of health conditions that can affect a woman's fertility—some you'd expect and some you wouldn't—and the medications you use to treat them can have bad effects, too, whether they're prescription or over the counter.

Medications are not tested for fertility effects before they go on the market and there's very little research done on this topic afterwards, so we don't know what many medications will do to your reproductive system. That said, here are some of the ones we know about that you may want to be aware of:

- **NSAIDs:** Prescription nonsteroidal anti-inflammatory drugs are used to treat rheumatologic conditions like arthritis. There have been several animal studies and at least three clinical studies showing that NSAIDs can cause luteinized unruptured follicle syndrome—which basically means that your egg matures but it never comes out of its follicle, so the sperm have nothing to fertilize when they show up at the rendezvous point wearing their spiffiest cologne. This seems to be limited to women who are taking NSAIDs for long periods, and it's reversible. There are several cases reported where infertile women who were on long-term courses of NSAIDs got pregnant after they stopped taking the medication. Over-the-counter NSAIDs are not known to have this effect.

- **THYROID MEDICATIONS:** Your thyroid medication levels need to be closely monitored to make sure that your thyroid hormones stay in the normal range. Those hormones are very important to ovulation and implantation, and the medications can throw you off.

- **DECONGESTANTS:** Using decongestants can dry up your cervical mucus, making it tough for the sperm to swim where they need to go. This is a temporary problem, though—don't worry about reducing your decongestants now if you're not going to try to get pregnant this week. Just try not to take any during your fertile windows when you're actually trying to conceive.

- **ANTIPSYCHOTIC MEDICATIONS:** Traditional antipsychotic medications and some of the newer antipsychotics block dopamine receptors and significantly increase levels of prolactin in the body, which can mess up your menstrual cycle and cause you to stop ovulating. "Well, that's irrelevant— I'm not psychotic," you say. But guess what? In addition to their use in treating schizophrenia and similar disorders, antipsychotics are also prescribed for several other conditions: insomnia, bipolar mood disorder, clinical depression and anxiety disorders. Sometimes, antipsychotics are prescribed along with SSRI inhibitors to boost the effectiveness of the antidepressants. One controversial report showed that sometimes, doctors don't tell their schizophrenic patients about the fertility effects because they figure it's better for them to be infertile.[1] If you're on an antipsychotic medication, ask if it's a first-generation or second-generation drug. The first-generation ones are more of a concern, but risperidone and paliperidone have also been shown to increase prolactin.[2]

- **ANTISEIZURE MEDICATIONS:** Medications for epilepsy are associated with infertility, and the more drugs you take, the worse the problem is—but it's not entirely clear whether it's the drugs or the epilepsy itself that causes infertility. Researchers did a study of 375 epileptic women in India and found that 7 percent of those who did not take any epilepsy drugs were infertile, as compared to 32 percent of those who took one epilepsy drug, 41 percent of those who took two epilepsy drugs and 60 percent of those who took three or more epilepsy drugs. The researchers suggested that it could be the medications having a cumulative effect, or it could just mean that the women who had to take more medications had more severe epilepsy, which is what caused the infertility. They also noted that phenobarbital was highly associated with infertility, whereas other drugs, such as valproate, were not.[3]

- **CANCER TREATMENTS:** Radiation and chemotherapy can both have bad effects on fertility, including causing early menopause. If the ovaries are anywhere near the path of radiation, eggs can get damaged—but there are also shields that can be used to block the ovaries in some cases, and it might be possible to temporarily move your ovaries out of the way by suturing them to the back of your uterus until treatments are over! Radiation

to the head can also interfere with hormone regulation.
The infertility effects from radiation may be temporary or permanent, which is one reason women may choose to freeze their eggs or embryos before cancer treatment. Chemotherapy drugs have differing effects on fertility, with some that are known to cause significant problems and some that aren't. Tamoxifen, a breast cancer medication that blocks estrogen, can cause endometrial polyps, which can interfere with fertility.

- **CYTOXAN:** This is a medication to treat lupus, and it can have detrimental effects on men's and women's fertility, particularly when it's taken long term.

- **DOMPERIDONE:** This is a medication to reduce nausea and vomiting associated with certain gastric disorders and to counteract the gastrointestinal effects of other medications. Some women have also used it to increase breast-milk production. However, it is not FDA-approved in the United States because of various risks (including the risk of cardiac arrest and sudden death), and one of the known side effects is that it can make you stop ovulating.

If you don't see a medication you take on this list, don't assume it's safe. The FDA assigns a category to every drug based on what it knows about its effects on pregnancy and birth. The categories are A, B, C, D and X. Here's what the categories mean:

A: In human studies, pregnant women used the medicine and their babies did not have any problems related to using the medicine.

B: In humans, there are no good studies. But in animal studies, pregnant animals received the medicine, and the babies did not show any problems related to the medicine.

Or

In animal studies, pregnant animals received the medicine, and some babies had problems. But in human studies, pregnant women used the medicine and their babies did not have any problems related to using the medicine.

C: In humans, there are no good studies. In animals, pregnant animals treated with the medicine had some babies with problems. However, sometimes the medicine may still help the human mothers and babies more than it might harm them.

Or

No animal studies have been done, and there are no good studies in pregnant women.

D: Studies in humans and other reports show that when pregnant women use the medicine, some babies are born with problems related to the medicine. However, in some serious situations, the medicine may still help the mother and the baby more than it might harm them.

X: Studies or reports in humans or animals show that mothers using the medicine during pregnancy may have babies with problems related to the medicine. There are no situations where the medicine can help the mother or baby enough to make the risk of problems worth it. These medicines should never be used by pregnant women.

When you're at the point of trying to conceive, follow those guidelines just as if you were already pregnant. Make sure that any dangerous medicines are out of your system before you get pregnant.

# Supplements and Herbs

Supplements can have a good, bad or neutral effect on your fertility and, again, most of them have never been tested in terms of fertility—

so be very cautious about what kinds of supplements you choose to put in your body. Here's our current roundup.

## The Good

- **IRON:** In a significant study done in 2006, researchers from Harvard found that women who took iron supplements were much less likely to have infertility that was caused by ovulatory dysfunction.[4]

- **FOLATE:** Folate is a form of vitamin B that occurs naturally in some foods and is added to others. It's essential for cell division and growth. You may know that you need extra folate while you're pregnant because it protects your baby from spina bifida and other neural-tube defects. It's important to start taking it at least three months before you plan to conceive because that's how long it takes to get the right levels in your body, and the baby's spinal cord develops right at the beginning of your pregnancy at a time when lots of women don't even know they're pregnant yet (and thus aren't taking prenatal vitamins).

In addition, there's now some suggestion that folate can also have a positive effect on fertility and improve the odds of success for infertility treatments. Make sure your multivitamin includes folate or just start taking prenatal vitamins during all your childbearing years as long as you're sexually active. There are no known downsides, so it's a good idea to take the supplement starting as soon as you start having sex, in case you ever have an unplanned pregnancy.

Being deficient in folate can also harm your fertility. Kyra had a genetic condition called MTHFR that made her folate-deficient, and she didn't even know it until she went for a second round of fertility testing. (More on MTHFR to come.)

NYU Fertility Center nutritionist Kim Ross suggests that if you need more than what's in your vitamin, take a supplement with the L-5-methyltetrahydrofolate (L-5-MTHF) form of folate, which is more bioavailable and soluble than folic acid. "It provides the all-natural form of folate and seems to help increase blood levels of folate better than folic acid," she says. It's available over the counter.

## Folate-Rich Foods

The RDA (Recommended Dietary Allowance) of folate when you're pregnant or trying to become pregnant is 600 mcg per day. You can meet your folate needs by eating folate-rich foods, such as . . .

| FOOD | DIETARY FOLATE EQUIVALENT (DFE) PER SERVING |
|---|---|
| Beef liver, braised, 3 ounces | 215 mcg |
| Spinach, boiled, ½ cup | 131 mcg |
| Black-eyed peas (cowpeas), boiled, ½ cup | 105 mcg |
| Breakfast cereals, fortified with 25% of the DV† | 100 mcg |
| Rice, white, medium-grain, cooked, ½ cup† | 90 mcg |
| Asparagus, boiled, 4 spears | 89 mcg |
| Spaghetti, cooked, enriched, ½ cup† | 83 mcg |
| Brussels sprouts, frozen, boiled, ½ cup | 78 mcg |
| Lettuce, romaine, shredded, 1 cup | 64 mcg |
| Avocado, raw, sliced, ½ cup | 59 mcg |

† Fortified with folic acid as part of the folate fortification program.

| FOOD | DIETARY FOLATE EQUIVALENT (DFE) PER SERVING |
|---|---|
| Spinach, raw, 1 cup | 58 mcg |
| Broccoli, chopped, frozen, cooked, ½ cup | 52 mcg |
| Mustard greens, chopped, frozen, boiled, ½ cup | 52 mcg |
| Green peas, frozen, boiled, ½ cup | 47 mcg |
| Kidney beans, canned, ½ cup | 46 mcg |
| Bread, white, 1 slice† | 43 mcg |
| Peanuts, dry roasted, 1 ounce | 41 mcg |
| Wheat germ, 2 tablespoons | 40 mcg |
| Tomato juice, canned, ¾ cup | 36 mcg |
| Crab, Dungeness, 3 ounces | 36 mcg |
| Orange juice, ¾ cup | 35 mcg |
| Turnip greens, frozen, boiled, ½ cup | 32 mcg |
| Orange, fresh, 1 small | 29 mcg |
| Papaya, raw, cubed, ½ cup | 27 mcg |

Source: Office of Dietary Supplements, National Institutes of Health

- **CoEnzyme Q-10 (CoQ10):** CoQ10 is an enzyme present in every healthy cell of your body. Your body makes it, and it fuels cells' mitochondria—the energy generator. As you age, your CoQ10 production goes down. Improving women's fertility is a fairly newly discovered possible benefit of CoQ10. It has been used to improve sperm parameters in men, but no one thought to try it for women's fertility. Then came an animal study that showed it improved fertility in mice, and

---

† Fortified with folic acid as part of the folate fortification program.

now researchers are working on human studies to see if the same results hold up. But it does make sense that it would—your egg is the biggest cell in your body and it needs a lot of energy. CoQ10 can help the egg make more energy.

- **SELENIUM:** Selenium is a mineral found in soil. You can get it from a variety of foods (seafood and Brazil nuts, in particular) or in supplement form. Numerous studies have pointed the finger at selenium deficiency when it comes to early miscarriage and infertility in both men and women. However, there haven't yet been any big trials to show how selenium supplementation might help fertility or prevent miscarriage.

## The Bad

In animal studies, high doses of the following supplements have been shown to harm fertility: St. John's wort (for depression), gingko biloba (for memory) and echinacea (for immune function). You don't need to stop taking them now if you're not trying to conceive, but stop at least three months before you plan to start trying—and that goes for your partner, too. These supplements may harm sperm as well as eggs.

There are other ingredients in herbal supplements that can act as natural pharmaceuticals, affecting your hormones. Don't think that just because something says herbal or all-natural, that means it's safe. In fact, it has the potential of being very unsafe because manufacturers don't even need to submit their products to the FDA for approval, meaning that they're just taken at their word about what's in the bottles. Talk to your doctor about everything you take. Bring the bottle (or a list of ingredients) to your next visit.

## The Pointless

There are many, many untested supplements offered for sale to people who are trying to get pregnant. Amazon currently lists 384 of them. Some of them have ingredients that at least may possibly be beneficial, but many of them are just plain useless. Don't bother buying stuff just because the internet says so. Know what you're spending your money on and what you're putting in your body. Ask your OB/GYN or fertility specialist about the ingredients in any supplement you're planning to try for fertility.

# Health Conditions That Can Reduce Your Fertility

## Endometriosis

If your periods hurt badly or it's painful to have sex, you might have endometriosis. This is a common condition (affecting 5–10 percent of women) in which the tissue that's supposed to line your uterus grows in places other than where it's supposed to; it may grow on the outside of your uterus, in or on your ovaries, on your intestines or bladder, or in your fallopian tubes. It can cause scar tissue to form and to inflame and distort the organs it affects. The American Society for Reproductive Medicine says that 30–50 percent of all infertile women have endometriosis.[5] It is not clear how endometriosis lowers fertility, whether it is mechanical, immunologic or it directly affects egg and sperm function, but IVF bypasses its ill effects.

How much it may affect your fertility depends on its severity— a mild case may have no effect, whereas a more severe case may prove insurmountable. There are several ways in which endometriosis can affect fertility: It may distort your reproductive organs; it may cause scarring and swelling, making it impossible for a fertilized egg to implant; and it may affect hormone levels. For women who are not trying to get pregnant, estrogen-blocking treatments may help ease symptoms, but, ultimately, surgical removal of endometriosis and scar tissue may be needed to treat infertility.

## Adenomyosis

Adenomyosis is something of a cousin to endometriosis. It's when endometrial tissue is found in muscle layers of your uterus. It affects about 1 percent of women in their lifetime, usually after age thirty-five and after they've already had children. Symptoms include prolonged, heavy menstrual bleeding; abdominal pain and bloating; an enlarged uterus; and severe menstrual cramps. Its effects on fertility are not yet clear; it's nowhere near as highly studied as endometriosis, but the limited data suggest that it can hinder fertility and have a negative effect on the outcome of IVF. Symptoms usually diminish or go away at perimenopause or menopause, and if there are painful symptoms, they may be treated with over-the-counter anti-inflammatory drugs or prescription NSAIDs. There are also hormone treatments and surgical treatments available for more severe cases. Traditionally, the only permanent solution for severe adenomyosis was hysterectomy, but there is now a procedure called adenomyomectomy that has been shown to preserve fertility in most cases.

## Fibroids

Fibroids are generally benign tumors growing in or around the uterus, and they're very common among women of childbearing age. It's highly likely that you have had one and don't even know it. Up to 75 percent of women will have fibroids at some point in their lives. In the majority of cases, they don't cause any symptoms, don't mess with your fertility and don't need to be treated. They typically either shrink or at least stop growing around menopause. But if they grow very large or if there are many of them, they can cause problems such as pressing on and distorting the fallopian tubes, or preventing an embryo from implanting. If that happens, they have to be removed, and the double-edged sword is that the surgery to remove them can also hinder your fertility.

A friend of Kyra's found out she had a tremendous fibroid in a very uncomfortable way:

*I knew I had a medium-sized fibroid (6 cm in circumference) when I was pregnant with my daughter. The OB/GYN kept an eye on it, but it didn't grow during the pregnancy and I forgot all about it afterwards. It didn't affect me for two years, but then I began having bladder problems here and there—incontinence when I'd laugh or exercise sometimes. I chalked it up to the terrible business of aging and didn't think much about it until the opposite problem occurred: One morning, I could not urinate at all. I had a full bladder and no way to release it—which was torture.*

*The fibroid had gotten so large that it closed off my bladder. I had to head to the ER for a catheter—and they told me I'd need surgery within the week, leaving me to run off and research surgeons. Most of the time, doctors compare tumor sizes to fruit— they'll tell you it's the size of a lemon or a grapefruit. They told me mine was the size of a baby's head. Creeptastic.*

*It made total sense now—I had been so frustrated that I had gained "belly weight" lately. I'd done a good job of losing the pregnancy weight quickly, but here I was two years later looking like I was pregnant again, with no explanation . . . well, my uterus had swollen out to the size of a five-month pregnancy from this fibroid intruder.*

*Because I wanted to preserve my fertility, that limited my options to a particular type of surgery called an abdominal myomectomy. Doctors explained that there was still a small risk of losing my fertility even with the myomectomy, but I'd have a much better chance than with the other recommended courses of action—like, for instance, hysterectomy! They also told me that my odds of retaining my fertility were also better with one large fibroid than with several smaller ones, and there is a smaller chance of recurrence that way, too.*

*I scared myself by reading some online horror stories about the procedure, but the aftereffects of the surgery were not painful for me. I felt weak and I walked funny for about two months afterwards—it is major abdominal surgery—but had no complications and didn't need anything stronger than Tylenol by the time I got home from the hospital. The surgeon didn't have to cut through my endometrium, which means that not only do I have a good chance of having retained my fertility, but it's even still possible for me to have another vaginal birth—normally, you need C-sections after going through an abdominal myomectomy because it's automatically considered a high-risk pregnancy.*

*All of my symptoms disappeared and I'm thrilled to say that I can go back to jumping around with my daughter and laughing my head off without worrying that I'm headed for an early trip down the adult diapers aisle.*

It's true that the large fibroids (above 6 cm) tend to cause the most problems, but that's not always the case. Some women with smaller fibroids have more symptoms—pain, abnormal bleeding, short menstrual cycles and infertility. This may be the case because there are many small fibroids, or it may just be that the fibroids are in bad spots.

Fibroids tend to grow during pregnancy because of all the additional hormones coursing through your body. Depending on size and placement, the fibroid could also interfere with the baby's development and nourishment. It's important to keep a close eye on fibroids before and during pregnancy, especially if you have any large ones.

One important thing to keep in mind is that if you do need surgery to remove a fibroid, choose a surgeon with extensive experience and a track record for not resorting to a hysterectomy. It's inevitable that a small portion of abdominal myomectomies will have to wind up as hysterectomies in emergency situations, but that should be a very small number. Some surgeons are quicker to resort to hysterectomy than others; ask what percentage of their myomectomies have turned into hysterectomies. Ten percent is too high. You want to hear that, out of hundreds of myomectomies they've performed, maybe one or two have needed to become hysterectomies.

Hysterectomies are simpler procedures; myomectomies can be complicated and require more skillful hands, so don't assume that your regular OB/GYN can handle it. You may want to look into a gynecological oncologist, because even though you are most likely not dealing with cancer, most of them have significant surgical experience, whereas OB/GYNs may do very few of these procedures.

And you don't need to wait very long after surgery to get pregnant. Depending on the type of procedure, Jamie says four to eight weeks afterwards is safe to start trying.

If you do discover that you have a small fibroid, don't panic! Remember that most of them will never need to be removed and will never cause problems.

## Uterine or Endometrial Polyps

Similar to fibroids, polyps are almost always benign growths. They're an overgrowth of the uterine lining (called the endometrium) and can cause bleeding in between periods or other abnormal menstrual bleeding. Polyps may be sessile (flat) or pedunculated (with a stalk), and the location can affect whether or not the polyp will interfere with your fertility. It's not possible for a doctor to know for sure whether a growth is a polyp or a fibroid until she actually removes it.

The risk of a polyp being malignant increases with age—particularly if you have postmenopausal bleeding. But in most cases, you won't even be aware that they exist; a doctor may spot them while doing a routine exam or during a workup for fertility treatments. The good news is that having polyps removed is now an outpatient procedure that doesn't require a D&C (dilation and curettage), which would mean scraping out the entire uterus and figuring that the polyps would be removed with the lining. Now doctors can use a microscopic morcellator that grabs only the abnormal tissue and grinds it up into a fine paste that is extracted by vacuum pressure. There is minimal tissue damage and no normal tissue is harmed, and the procedure can take mere minutes.

The risks involved in this procedure are minimal (as with any kind of surgery like this, there is a small risk of infection, bleeding, perforation of the uterus and scarring) and you should be discharged within about two hours. The polyps will be tested to make sure they're not cancerous, any abnormal bleeding you may have had should stop and your probability of getting pregnant should improve. You can start trying to conceive one month after the procedure.

One of Jamie's patients, Denise, had several polyps when she came to the clinic.

"I can't guarantee this is what's causing your infertility," he said, "But I think it might be. So we have two options: Remove them now and take that out of the equation, or try IVF first and wait and see."

There was no single right answer because women with polyps certainly do get pregnant sometimes, and it's not possible to know with any degree of certainty which ones will have problems and which ones won't. But she elected to have the surgery, had no complications and was pregnant two months later.

It's important for patients to understand what their doctor knows and doesn't know and what their options are so they can make educated decisions. Never be afraid to ask questions if you've been diagnosed with polyps or anything else—if a doctor doesn't want to spend time explaining what your options are and how things may affect you, then find a new doctor. You deserve to be in charge of your body and an active participant in your own care.

## Migraines

Migraines themselves are not known to have any effect on fertility; however, they can be a predictor of endometriosis. If you get migraines, you're more than twice as likely to also have endometriosis. Get checked out.

## Diabetes

Both type 1 and type 2 diabetes can have negative effects on fertility and on sustaining a pregnancy. Diabetes can mess with your periods and send you into early menopause, among other problems. There was a time when diabetic women were advised not to get pregnant, but nowadays, if you can keep your diabetes under control with medication and diet, fertility rates are close to normal.

## Polycystic Ovary Syndrome

Affecting about 10 percent of women, polycystic ovary syndrome (PCOS) can be a serious pain in the butt. It's a mysterious condition in which you get a bunch of cysts on your ovaries and your hormones go all out of whack. Normally, your ovaries produce a small amount of male hormones (androgens), but when you have PCOS, your body produces too much of these substances. It can cause a whole range of not-very-fun symptoms, including acne, weight gain, hair thinning on your head, hair growing on your face and body, and depression. And, of course, it can also mess up your periods and your fertility. You may ovulate much more sporadically or not at all. You may also need fertility medications to help you get pregnant.

It's really important to exercise and keep your weight under control if you have PCOS. One of the earmarks of this syndrome is insulin resistance: when cells stop using insulin properly, leading the pancreas to make more and more insulin to try to make up for its ineffectiveness. The cells then have problems absorbing glucose and converting it to energy, so there's an abundance of glucose floating around in the bloodstream that then turns to fat. People with PCOS often develop type 2 diabetes and cardiac problems.

This insulin resistance is sometimes treated with insulin-sensitizing agents or steroids, but the primary way to treat it is through diet and exercise. Belly fat is seen as a major contributing factor to insulin resistance, and a sedentary lifestyle makes the problem worse. Exercise helps your body in so many ways, but one of them is to improve your sensitivity to insulin and to burn off excess glucose. When you build muscle, you're also building a glucose-burning factory that can reverse the effects of PCOS and make you more fertile. If you're not ovulating, even just minor weight loss can help you start again.

## Pituitary Tumors

About 20 percent of the population has one or more pituitary tumors. The pituitary gland is a pea-sized structure at the base of your brain that releases hormones, and tumors there are rarely cancerous or symptomatic. However, when a pituitary tumor does cause symptoms, those symptoms may include hyperthyroidism, Cushing's disease and hyperprolactinemia, all three of which can cause infertility.

## Cushing's Disease and Cushing's Syndrome

This is a rare condition where there is too much cortisol in the body, normally due to long-term or excessive use of the steroid medications known as glucocorticoids (most commonly, prednisone, prednisolone and dexamethasone). These steroids have anti-inflammatory properties and doctors prescribe them for a variety of conditions, including asthma, allergies, postsurgical inflammation, arthritis and cancer pain. Inhaled corticosteroids for asthma are less dangerous because they stay in the airway; very little gets into the rest of the body.

Cushing's syndrome can also be caused by problems within your body, primarily tumors that give off cortisol or a related hormone called ACTH. When the tumor causing it is in the pituitary gland, it's called Cushing's disease instead of Cushing's syndrome.

Most people with Cushing's have a red, round face ("moon face"), with obesity above the waist but thin arms and legs. It can cause a variety of symptoms, but infertility is a major one. Women with Cushing's often have irregular periods, or none at all, and very seldom get pregnant. Men with Cushing's may also develop infertility and decreased sex drive. The condition is often treatable, however, by addressing the underlying issue—reducing or stopping steroids, or surgery or medication to address tumors. Stay aware of the symptoms if you're on long-term or high doses of glucocorticoids. If you suspect Cushing's, check with your doctor before stopping your prescription. Fertility normally returns once Cushing's is no longer active.

## Hyperprolactinemia

Your pituitary gland, which sits in the base of your brain, produces a hormone called prolactin. Normally, it produces just a small amount, then it produces a lot when you're pregnant and breast-feeding. It's the hormone that controls a woman's milk supply. However, sometimes women who aren't pregnant have abnormally high levels of prolactin floating around, and that causes problems with the menstrual cycle and fertility. Often the cause is a tumor on the pituitary gland that's either secreting prolactin or collapsing the gland and preventing it from getting signals to stop producing the hormone. This may be treated with medications (or stopping certain medications, such as antipsychotics, that may be causing the problem) or surgery.

## Hirsutism

Do you have thick hair growing on your chin or abdomen? Could you potentially grow a little beard if you didn't keep it under control? Then you likely have hirsutism, a condition in which there is excessive hair growth on women's faces and bodies. (The hair may also be growing on your chest, back, toes, upper lip, etc., but hair growth on the chin and abdomen are the most frequent indicators.) This is a giant tip-off that you have an androgen excess—that is, that your body is producing too much testosterone. Excess testosterone alone can cause problems with your fertility; in addition, it's also strongly associated with PCOS and insulin resistance. Hirsutism is also highly genetic—if women in your family have the condition, you're at much higher risk of having it, too.

## Bacterial Vaginosis

This itchy problem can be the result of bubble baths or other situations where bacteria get inside the vagina. You're at higher risk for it if you smoke or douche. It's a very common infection that usually resolves on its own in just a few days, but if it doesn't, then antibiotics can clear it up. It hasn't been shown to have any effect on conception, but it's associated with a twofold greater risk of miscarriage in the first trimester—so be sure to get checked out if you have vaginal itch or discomfort when you're trying to conceive or you're pregnant.

## Thyroid Problems

Whether your thyroid is overactive (hyperthyroidism) or underactive (hypothyroidism), it can affect your fertility. It can cause irregular menstrual cycles and miscarriage as well.

Jamie has treated several patients with previously unexplained infertility who turned out to simply need thyroid medication—which is safe to take while pregnant (in fact, you have to increase your dose during pregnancy, but, as noted earlier, the medication needs to be closely monitored). Hypothyroidism can cause weight gain, constipation, lethargy and cold extremities. Hyperthyroidism is often associated with weight loss, difficulty sleeping and jittery feelings. However, most cases are subclinical, meaning that they don't show symptoms.

They're among the many conditions that often show up first during a fertility workup by doing routine bloodwork. Meredith, one of Jamie's recent patients, had an irregular menstrual cycle and had recently lost ten pounds, so he sent her to an endocrinologist and found out she had Graves' disease—an autoimmune disorder that causes your body to attack the thyroid. It initially causes hyperthyroidism and is commonly associated with a telling feature—bulging eyes (though that's not always present)—and may also be associated with anxiety, rapid heartbeat, tremors, sensitivity to heat, diarrhea, enlarged thyroid gland and skin changes. It causes ovulatory dysfunction that's a protective mechanism against getting pregnant with the disease—you don't want to get pregnant with Graves' disease or you'll most likely miscarry. Meredith is now getting treatment for her disorder before trying to get pregnant again.

## Sleep Disorders

Several sleep disorders can disrupt your hormones, and therefore your fertility. Any kind of disorder where you're not getting enough quality sleep can throw off your hormone balance. This includes common problems, such as insomnia, sleep apnea and restless legs syndrome. Sleep apnea may also lead to insulin resistance, which in turn decreases fertility.

## Gum Disease

"What? What does my mouth have to do with my fertility?" We know, it's a weird one, but researchers recently determined that people with gum disease (which is about 10–20 percent of the population) take longer to get pregnant—two months longer, on average, and the effect is more pronounced on non-Caucasian women.[6] So keep up your flossing and get those regular cleanings!

## Inflammatory Bowel Disease

Crohn's disease and ulcerative colitis have a minor impact on fertility. If you're not having an active episode and you haven't had an ileostomy, you should be fine. When the disease is flaring up, both men's and women's fertility can be compromised. Sperm counts are lower and so are conception rates.

## Down Syndrome

All men and most women with Down syndrome are infertile.

## Mayer-Rokitansky-Küster-Hauser Syndrome

This is a condition where a woman is born without a uterus. She still has functioning ovaries, but no uterus to carry a baby. At this time, her options would be limited to surrogacy or adoption.

## Gastroschisis

This is a rare condition where there's a hole in a baby's abdominal cavity and his or her intestines are sticking out at birth. It requires surgery within the first few days after birth to fix, and because of that, there may be scar tissue or permanent damage to the reproductive organs. The condition is more common when the baby's mother is a teenager or if she smokes or drinks during pregnancy. Most people who have had gastroschisis don't have a belly button, but instead have a scar in its place.

## MTHFR Genetic Mutation

The MTHFR (methylenetetrahydrofolate reductase) gene helps make an enzyme to process amino acids, and those who have mutations of this gene (there are several types) have an impaired ability to metabolize folic acid. It's very common—at least 20 percent of the population has one copy of the mutation and up to 14 percent have two copies of the mutation. The various types of mutations can affect people in different ways and can be symptomatic or asymptomatic, but one of the things it's known for is being associated with recurrent miscarriages and a slightly higher risk of neural-tube defects. You can find out if you have this genetic mutation through a simple blood test. Jamie recommends that women with MTHFR mutations take extra folic acid when they're ready to conceive.

Doctors didn't know anything about this gene until the Human Genome Project in 2003, so it's a newly identified factor in infertility and it's not yet clear how much of an effect it has (on fertility or anything else). But considering that the treatment for it is so easy, Jamie says that it's a no-brainer: Folic acid is a nontoxic, water-soluble vitamin with no downsides, so he says it's not a hard decision to take an extra 2–3 mg.

### Kyra Says . . .

I'm one of those people with the MTHFR mutation. After two rounds of embryo transfers that ended in disappointing miscarriages, I took the blood test for MTHFR, which showed I had a single mutation. My fertility team bumped up my folic acid intake by an extra milligram. The next transfer, whammo! I got pregnant with twins, and this time it held. With more folate circulating in my system, I was a babymaking dynamo! And there was a side benefit—it would greatly reduce the chances that either of my babies would be born with a neural-tube defect. It was a win-win all around.

## Structural Abnormalities

There are several possible uterine abnormalities, but only some of them seem to affect fertility.

## Septate Uterus

This is what it's called when there's a muscular or fibrous wall (called a "septate") that divides the uterus roughly in half. The wall may be present in only part of the uterus ("incomplete septate") or the whole length of the uterus ("complete septate"). This may be discovered during a routine exam, but is more likely to be found only when you're seeking treatment for infertility or recurrent miscarriages. Outpatient surgery can remove the septate and restore fertility and normal pregnancy outcomes in most cases.

## Bicornate Uterus

This is a heart-shaped uterus that has two "horns." When the uterus is being formed in a fetus, it does start out with two separate horns that eventually are meant to fuse together—but sometimes that doesn't happen. This condition can lead to premature labor and other pregnancy problems. There is limited data about the surgery to correct this condition, but what's out there does suggest that it can be successfully corrected and lead to normal pregnancy outcomes.

## Unicornate Uterus

This condition occurs when the uterus has just one horn and one fallopian tube and is about half the size it should be. There is often also a second, smaller horn that is unconnected and noncommunicative to the uterus. There is no surgery to correct this problem (other than to remove the noncommunicative horn, which is a good idea because if pregnancy occurs there, it's as dangerous as an ectopic pregnancy). Successful pregnancy is possible, but fertility is reduced because of the single fallopian tube, and pregnancy outcomes are often not good because the uterus is so small and malformed. This is an extremely rare condition, affecting about one in four thousand women.

## Double Uterus

It is also possible to have two separate uteri. Each one may have its own cervix and even its own vagina (yes, some women have two vaginas!), or the two uteruses may share an opening. This is not typically a problem with fertility, but pregnancies are automatically categorized as high-risk because the uteruses are half-size and there's a higher risk of a condition known as incompetent cervix (a cervix that opens too soon because of the baby's weight pressing on it). Surgery is rarely recommended unless it's needed to save a fetus's life. Again, this is a condition you may not realize you have until you are either pregnant and at a prenatal exam or going for infertility treatment.

## Retroverted Uterus

Also known as a tipped, tilted or backward uterus, this refers to the normal variation where a woman's uterus is tilted backward toward her spine instead of forward. About 20 percent of all women have a retroverted uterus. It's not normally a big deal and rarely causes symptoms (pain during sex and pelvic exams, primarily). Sometimes it happens after childbirth and then corrects itself within a few months. It is not usually a factor in fertility, but in cases of unexplained infertility, doctors may speculate that it's the problem.

## Relax: Don't Worry about These

Here are a few health conditions and medications you might think would affect your fertility, but they've never been shown to:

- Yeast infections
- Urinary tract infections (as long as you treat them before they get out of control)
- Toxic shock syndrome (which can kill you—but assuming it doesn't . . . )
- High blood pressure
- Antidepressant medications
- Asthma and seasonal allergies
- Oxycodone

We're still learning about the many causes of infertility, which is why there are so many cases where the cause is unknown. The good news is that most of these causes of infertility are treatable or reversible once they're identified.

Chapter 6

# Don't Drink That,
# Put Down That Lipstick and
# Change Your Shower Curtain

## The Chemicals in Our Lives

While modern science has given us all kinds of amazing advances in the
medical field, it is also responsible for some of the worst disasters of our
time, like the truly frightening things happening in our environment—
radioactive leaks at nuclear plants, global warming, landfills overflowing
with junk that will never break down, the list goes on and on.

We have more medications and tests and treatments at our disposal
than ever, but we also have more toxic, unnatural things all around us
that are making us sick. We are being bombarded by bad stuff in our
environment every day, and we're just learning in bits and pieces how
all that bad stuff is affecting us. It can be a vicious cycle of "Take this to
treat what that other thing did to you. Now take this to treat the side
effects from the other medication. Now take this to treat the problems
from the third medication..."

Don't assume that the government or anyone else is protecting
you, and that manufacturers wouldn't be allowed to sell really toxic
stuff. It just isn't true. For many years, doctors were allowed to prescribe cocaine for people's "nerves," Coca-Cola once contained cocaine

and cigarettes were marketed practically as a health supplement. In most cases, it takes years and years of massive proof for the government to step in and ban a harmful product.

One of the biggest environmental safety issues of this decade has been the recognition that certain plastics and chemicals used in our everyday lives have been screwing up our babies and ourselves.

# BPA

BPA (Bisphenol-A) is an industrial chemical that's used in a load of products from plastic containers to tooth sealants to soup cans. It's used to harden polycarbonate plastics (as in water bottles) and to make epoxy resins that line food and beverage containers. In 1996 and 1997, scientists published reports showing that even ridiculously tiny amounts of BPA had a major effect on mice in many ways—particularly their reproductive organs—which drew a lot of attention in the scientific community. The plastics industry freaked out about being exposed like this and funded two studies in response to show that BPA was safe. Of course, there was a conflict of interest in these studies.

BPA mimics estrogen. Our bodies can't tell the difference between it and estradiol, one of the three major estrogens. BPA can bind with estrogen receptors and disrupt the way our hormones naturally work. Manufacturers have said that it would have to be present at very high levels to cause any bad effects on humans, whereas some researchers said that it caused permanent health effects even at very low levels.

As with many things, the truth is probably somewhere in the middle. We're all doing the best we can with the information we have at the time, and none of us knew anything about BPA before these reports. While it doesn't look as though BPA is good for you, it also doesn't look as though it's the most terrible substance known to humanity, so don't beat yourself up over the things you've already done "wrong." We're providing the following information because we think it's important enough for you to think about and know, but not because we want you to panic.

In 2007, the National Institute of Environmental Health Sciences (NIEHS) organized a meeting of scientists from the United States, Germany and Japan from a variety of disciplines to discuss what they knew about BPA, what they suspected and what was still unknown. Afterwards, the attendees published a report about their conclusions. Some of the most salient points were as follows:

- **BPA IS WIDESPREAD.** Because the chemical leaches out of plastic and can linings under normal use, it's present in our food supply, in our water and in our air. It's found at detectable levels in the bloodstream of 95 percent of all the people researchers tested. In fact, it's so widespread that it's found in most *fetuses*. That's right—you probably already had BPA in your bloodstream before you were born because your mother had it in hers while you were developing. It's also found in breast milk.

- **OUR BODIES' SENSITIVITY TO ENDOCRINE DISRUPTORS** such as BPA is different at different life stages—we may be more affected by a chemical like this at times when crucial systems are still developing, which means that the time before birth and shortly after birth are extra-sensitive times. The scientists determined that when BPA was administered to lab animals as fetuses or newborns, the result was organizational changes in their prostate, breast, testis, mammary glands, body size, brain structure and chemistry, and behavior.

- **PREGNANT MICE AND RATS EXPOSED TO BPA** were giving birth to males with low sperm counts and low testosterone secretions. The females went into puberty early. The "BPA babies" grew larger and had more hyperactive behaviors. Liver enzymes were disrupted as well.

Soon after this meeting, the media began educating people about the potential dangers and prevalence of BPA, especially in baby products. It wasn't until 2012 that the FDA formally banned its use in baby bottles and sippy cups, and that's only because the plastics industry actually asked them to! They'd nearly all stopped using BPA in those specific products by then anyway, and they wanted to eliminate confusion so people wouldn't keep asking if particular products were BPA-free or not.

It's great that it's no longer in baby bottles or sippy cups, but BPA is still being used in plastic water bottles and water cooler jugs, canned foods, dental sealants and even the coatings on receipts. And researchers have found trace amounts in all sorts of paper products, from money to toilet paper, paper towels, business cards and newspapers.

One of the problems is that it's effective at what it does—in canned foods, spraying on a coating of BPA in the lining greatly reduces the chance that the food inside will spoil. As of now, manufacturers haven't found another substance that works as well, and they probably won't unless we make a lot more noise to say that we're not going to consume canned goods with BPA anymore. Financial pressure—voting with our wallets—is what made the baby-product manufacturers change their tune. Drying up the demand for canned goods until they find a safer alternative means that they'll hustle to find a safer alternative.

But to get to that point, we need to understand that the evidence has been growing. We're learning that BPA may have even more negative effects than scientists recognized just a few years ago. One newer finding is that there is an association between BPA and human infertility and miscarriage rates—not shocking, considering we already saw this in animal studies. Back in 2002, a study showed that male mice that ingested BPA had trouble getting their lady mice pregnant.[1]

Then in 2012, a study of 170 women from China showed that the women with high levels of serum BPA had a higher rate of miscarriage. The levels of BPA were even higher among women who'd had several unexplained miscarriages.[2] A second study by a team in the United States showed that women with the highest levels of BPA in their blood had an 80 percent higher chance of miscarriage than the women with the lowest levels.[3]

## Jamie Says . . .

"Association" is not the same as "causation." We have to be careful to note that when a study shows that there is an association between two things—in this case, BPA and infertility and miscarriage—it doesn't necessarily mean that BPA caused the infertility or miscarriages. There is still a chance that there's another factor (or factors) at play, or even that it's a coincidence. These are also all relatively small studies. But due to the growing evidence, my advice is still to steer clear of BPA as much as possible.

## Tips for Avoiding BPA

- Don't leave plastic water bottles in the heat. Heating the plastic causes it to leach BPA into the water at much higher concentrations. If you accidentally left your water bottle in the car on a hot day, throw it out.

- Use stainless steel or BPA-free plastic reusable water bottles.

- Whenever possible, get e-mail receipts instead of printed receipts. Wash your hands after handling printed receipts.

- Avoid canned goods as much as you can, particularly soup and other "wet" canned food, which has the highest BPA concentration.

- Don't microwave anything in a plastic container. If you eat a frozen dinner, put it on a plate before heating.

- Don't put boiling or very hot liquid into plastic containers that contain BPA.

- Get rid of old food storage containers. Tupperware manufactured since March 2010 is BPA-free. Rubbermaid since January 2010 is also BPA-free, and there's a helpful page here that shows pictures of which of their previous products contained BPA: www.rubbermaid.com/Pages/LearnAboutBPA.aspx.

- Limit your cleaning and reuse of BPA-containing food containers; if you're not sure of the BPA status of a plastic mug or plate, for instance, don't scrub it with an abrasive sponge or expose it to the dishwasher, which can release more BPA. Hand-wash gently.

- Bring your own cup/thermos/stainless steel water bottle to parties and events where it's likely that they'll serve you in a plastic cup.

- Drink beer and soda from glass bottles instead of cans.

# The Downside to Information

We'd like to reiterate Jamie's advice—you can make yourself crazy trying to research and do everything exactly right. Some people feel comforted when they research the heck out of something and feel as if they're more in control, but if it hits a point where you're feeling anxious and stressed and guilty about the choices you've made, then it's probably time to step back and relax. Remind yourself of all the mistakes your parents made with you. You're not dead yet. There, feel better?

# Pfft to Phthalates

While BPA has been a bigger buzzword in recent years, phthalates (pronounced thā-lates) stink, too.

They're a group of about twenty-five human-made chemicals that are used to make some plastics more flexible or bendable and harder to break, and they're also used as dyes, solvents and adhesives. And, like BPA, phthalates are all over the place. They're in vinyl flooring, food packaging, your raincoat, plastic bags, lots of cleaning products, cosmetics, air fresheners, shower curtains, lunch bags, garden hoses, hairspray, shoes, steering wheels, erasers, toothbrushes, binders, artificial Christmas trees, plastic wrap and probably in your soil. Luckily, phthalates bind with soil, so they rarely get into the groundwater supply, but that's a small consolation. Have we mentioned they're also in many sex toys? Aw, man!

Our body's endocrine system secretes hormones into our bloodstream, and phthalates are in the category known as endocrine disruptors. They block androgens (male hormones) and can affect both male and female reproductive systems.

Phthalates can enter your body through your digestive system when you eat or drink something that's been tainted with the chemical, they can enter through your skin, you can inhale them or you can even get them intravenously (medical tubing usually contains phthalates). They don't stay put in the products they're in—in other words, just because you can't see the phthalates jumping out of the shower curtain while you're in there taking a nice, long steamy one doesn't mean they're not floating into the air while you're in there. They are.

Our bodies are capable of metabolizing and excreting phthalates, so they don't just keep building up, but we have an ongoing stream of exposure in our daily lives. Just a few years ago, scientists discovered that parents were unwittingly giving their babies phthalates when they used baby powder, lotion or baby shampoo—the phthalates from the packaging were absorbed in the powder, lotion and shampoo and then applied to the baby's skin and absorbed into the bloodstream.

Also, like BPA, there have been lots of animal studies of phthalates, but human studies of these chemicals have been small and few. The Environmental Protection Agency (EPA) has expressed concern about phthalates "because of their toxicity and the evidence of pervasive human and environmental exposure to these chemicals."

Human studies have shown links between phthalate exposure and lowered sperm counts, atopic dermatitis in children and asthma. Animal studies have revealed links between phthalate exposure and early onset of puberty, hampered male reproductive tract development, reproductive and genital defects, hormone abnormalities, miscarriage, lowered testosterone and lowered sperm counts.

One interesting study tested whether or not polyvinyl chloride (PVC) flooring in the home had any effect on young children developing asthma. Sure enough, kids who had PVC flooring in their bedrooms did get asthma more often than kids without—but that's not the interesting part. What surprised the researchers was that it was even more likely for kids to get asthma if the PVC flooring was in their parents' bedroom, leading the researchers to theorize that the more important time for exposure was in the womb.[4] Could it be that a woman sleeping in a room with PVC floors while pregnant led to the child developing asthma years later? We can't say for sure, but that's what the researchers believe—and it is feasible.

On *60 Minutes,* pediatric urologist Dr. Harold Snyder said he thinks exposure to chemicals such as phthalates during pregnancy are responsible for the sharp increases in male sex organ birth defects over the past thirty to forty years, including a threefold increase in hypospadias—where the opening of the urethra is on the bottom of the penis instead of at the tip, so the pee dribbles out the wrong spot. There's also been a twofold increase in undescended testicles, and some scientists are also now warning of a "sperm count crisis"; according to several published studies, sperm counts in many countries are on the decline.

Surely, phthalates are not the only cause of these problems. It's not even 100 percent certain that they're part of the problem, but, again, as with BPA, the evidence is strong, and it doesn't hurt to make changes where you can.

# It's Not on the Label

You're not going to find phthalates on an ingredients label. In some cases, you'll find the opposite: a product that declares it's *PVC-free* or *phthalate-free* on its packaging. That's helpful! Otherwise, you have no idea what's hidden by one ugly little word that appears almost ubiquitously on cosmetic and cleaning-product packaging: *fragrance.* That little label hides myriad sins.

Here's what's even worse: You might find products that are labeled *BPA-free* and be tricked into thinking they're safe—when, in fact, they never contained BPA but they're chock-full of phthalates and other screwy chemicals.

# The Alternatives

When the government banned certain phthalates from kids' toys, that didn't mean that manufacturers would just remove them and not substitute something else. Companies are not required to disclose what chemicals they use in manufacturing, so they could choose alternates to phthalates that are known to be even more dangerous—or chemicals that are completely untested—and not tell anybody. It's like the honor system . . . and corporations are not always honorable.

California Environmental Protection Agency toxicologist Stephen Dizio said on National Public Radio (NPR), "There are 80,000 chemicals in commerce. We know something about [the] toxicity of about 400 of them. That really means that things come and go in the marketplace that you have no idea what will happen."

# How to Identify Plastics to Avoid

It's not possible to live a phthalate- or BPA-free life in modern society, but you can make a dent in how prevalent they are in your life. Pay attention to the products you use and buy and see how many you can replace with safer alternatives. Use tin foil instead of plastic wrap when storing leftovers, for instance, and use a PVC-free shower curtain. When you must use plastics, pay attention to their recycling numbers.

On the bottom of plastic containers, there is a number inside the triangular recycling symbol. Numbers 1, 2, 4 and 5 indicate that the packaging has no known significantly bad effects on health. Luckily, 1 is the most common for drink bottles. It's polyethylene terephthalate, abbreviated PET or PETE, and it has a low risk of leaching chemicals unless you heat it up.

The ones to watch out for are labeled 3, 6 and 7. The number 3 stands for vinyl and PVC, which are likely to contain phthalates. The number 6 is for polystyrene, which can be made into hard plastic or foam products, best known as Styrofoam. It's used plenty with food—in take-out containers, in disposable cups for hot drinks, disposable plates and so on. Unfortunately, it shouldn't be. There's evidence that it leaches toxic chemicals into food and drinks. Lots of people know it's bad for the environment because it releases harmful crap during its manufacture and can't readily be recycled, but now you know it could harm your health and fertility, too.

Number 7 stands for "other." It's a catchall term for all the types of plastics that don't fit into the other categories. Some are considered safe, while others are toxic. Polycarbonate is in this category, and that's the one that contains BPA. So if you see the number 7, the item may or may not contain BPA—you'd have to research further to find out. But if you have the option to pick something that doesn't have one of the "dangerous numbers," then do it.

Be aware, too, that many items use different kinds of plastics. When researching breast pumps, a friend of mine realized that even if the pump itself was made of a "safe" plastic, often the tubing, valves or other components weren't.

# The Price of That Nice Scent

We mentioned that air fresheners contain phthalates, but to compound the problem, aerosols contain VOCs (volatile organic compounds) that can cause problems with fertility and compromise the health of a fetus. Think about all the aerosol products you may use: glass cleaner, wood cleaner, deodorant, hairspray, canned air duster, perfume, disinfectant, nail polish dryer, spray paint and the like.

Cut down on them as much as possible and switch to safer alternatives. Vinegar is a powerful and versatile cleaning agent, and there are several pump-spray cleaners with all-natural cleansers. When deodorizing a room, try using baking soda or Borax rather than spraying chemicals into the air. Switch to roll-on deodorants and spritz perfumes instead of aerosol versions.

And although candles don't contain aerosol, most of them still *do* give off VOCs. Most candles are made from paraffin, and when scientists studied the gases they emit, they found a range of chemicals that could rival the toxicity of cigarette smoke. Unscented soy candles, however, didn't give off VOCs.

Lead researcher Dr. Ruhullah Massoudi, a chemistry professor at the University of South Carolina, says, "For a person who lights a candle every day for years or just uses them frequently, inhalation of these dangerous pollutants drifting in the air could contribute to the development of health risks like cancer, common allergies and even asthma. None of the vegetable-based candles produce toxic chemicals."

To lower the risk of VOCs from your candles, use soy-based or beeswax candles (they are more expensive; you can find them at health food stores). If you're going to use traditional paraffin candles, use them in well-ventilated spaces, opt for thin wicks and keep your exposure to a minimum.

# Parabens

Parabens are another group of chemicals used as preservatives in lots of cosmetics, foods, toiletries and medicines. They're good at killing bacteria and fungi, so they're widely used—and preservatives are necessary even in cosmetics to make sure you don't get infections. You'll most often see parabens in ingredients lists as methylparaben, ethylparaben, propylparaben, butylparaben, isobutylparaben, isopropylparaben and benzylparaben.

Along with acting as preservatives, they also have weak estrogenic properties, meaning that they mimic the estrogen you produce naturally and confuse your body.

Until recently, parabens were thought of as perfectly safe. They rarely cause allergic reactions (rashes), have no scent and have been used extensively since the 1930s. But in the early 2000s, animal studies revealed the estrogenlike effect. It's also been theorized that parabens harm male fertility, but again, studies are inconsistent. Some have said that parabens are associated with lower sperm counts, whereas others don't show any association. One study said that only a particular type of paraben—butylparaben—was associated with sperm DNA damage.

It's difficult to analyze the true long-term health effects of parabens (and any other groups of chemicals) because we're all exposed to multiple types of parabens every day. It's hard to have a control group in a scientific experiment when you really can't prevent people's exposure to these chemicals "in the wild." It's also impossible to measure the cumulative effect of different parabens over time—many studies have looked at individual parabens in limited-time doses.

One recent small study examined the paraben levels in the urine of fertility patients and checked to see if women with higher levels of various parabens had lower ovarian reserves. For the most part, they didn't. Only one type of paraben (propylparaben) was associated with lower ovarian reserves, and the researchers said that further studies should be done to confirm if there's really a connection.[5]

But considering that we know parabens are easily absorbed in the skin and considering that we know they have estrogenlike properties (which can be a contributing factor for both breast cancer and infertility), it's worth considering limiting your use of parabens as much as possible.

# Lead in Lipstick

In 2007, the Campaign for Safe Cosmetics released a report called "A Poison Kiss: The Problem of Lead in Lipstick." In it, the report's authors explained that they had hired an independent laboratory to test thirty-three red lipsticks bought at stores across the United States—and that two-thirds of the lipsticks tested contained lead.

You probably already know that lead is bad news. It's a powerful neurotoxin, and lead poisoning can lead to serious problems for children: lowered IQs, behavioral problems, kidney and nerve dysfunction, seizures, headaches, nausea, learning disabilities and a range of other symptoms—up to and including death. Typically, lead poisoning in children has been associated with peeling lead-based paint. (Lead is no longer used in household paint, but it was until 1978, which means that it's still present in most homes built before then.)

Lead can be ingested or inhaled, and it isn't good for anyone, but it's particularly dangerous for kids age six and under and for pregnant women because lead can cross the placenta and affect the fetus. It's something to watch out for in your childbearing years before you get pregnant, too, because you don't want to have high lead levels built up in your system when you do start trying to have a baby. High lead levels have been shown to have a negative effect on both men's and women's fertility, and are associated with higher rates of miscarriage.

Lead doesn't break down in the body; it just stays there and accumulates over the years. There is no such thing as a "safe" level of lead. We still don't even know all the health problems that lead can cause, or why some people are affected by fairly low levels of lead while others can withstand higher levels. It's a roll of the dice that you don't want to take if you can avoid it, so one place you certainly don't want lead is in your lipstick.

As of now, the FDA has done nothing in response to the proof of lead in lipsticks. Currently, a manufacturer could sell you a lipstick made entirely of lead and that would be legal.

## How to Deal with Lead in Lipstick

So what can you do about it?

First, don't assume that the more expensive brands are better. In fact, the brand that ranked the best in the FDA's study was Wet 'n' Wild, the super-discount brand you can find on endcaps at drugstores for about $1 per lipstick. And even more telling, don't assume that because a brand is known for being "eco-friendly" or "natural" that it's lead-free. Burt's Bees was one of the worst-ranked brands. Their toffee lip shimmer contained a lead content of 2.81 parts per million. And when it came to some brands, like Avon, the lead level depended entirely on the color—some did well and others didn't.

Read the full FDA results here: www.fda.gov/cosmetics/products-ingredients/products/ucm137224.htm#expanalyses. You'll find a list of four hundred lipsticks and how well they did. Our advice is to stick to lipsticks that fared well on the test if you're going to wear lipstick at all.

You have a better chance of having no lead if you choose colorless lip balms and glosses rather than lipstick. For instance, Vaseline Lip Therapy Lip Balm gets the best possible rating (0) from the Skin Deep Cosmetics Database.

You can also make sure to blot your lipstick so you don't wind up swallowing any excess, wear it sparingly and remove it before you eat or go to sleep.

Finally, you can lend your voice to the chorus of those urging the FDA to put limits on the amount of lead allowed in cosmetics. History has shown that consumer pressure often prompts the FDA to finally make a move.

## Other Sources of Lead

In addition to lipstick and peeling paint, here are other places you can encounter lead:

- Toys made outside the United States
- Pottery and ceramic tableware, especially terra-cotta dishes and pots from Mexico
- Vinyl miniblinds manufactured before 1998 and imported from China, Indonesia, Taiwan and Mexico (see the warning here: www.cchealth.org/lead-poison/pdf/miniblinds.pdf)
- Fishing sinkers (usually made entirely of lead)
- Christmas lights
- Soil
- Costume jewelry
- Artificial turf
- Rubber playground surfaces
- Plumbing pipes
- Solder (plumbers may still use lead solder to connect copper pipes)
- Imported candies
- Bullets
- Batteries
- Radiators
- Leaded crystal (glasses, vases, beads, etc.)

# Toluene, Benzene and Other Solvents

Toluene is an organic solvent that has been shown in several studies to be associated with lowered fertility. In one study of women who worked in a German printing company (toluene is the only solvent used there), it took women twice as long, on average, to get pregnant if they had daily exposure to toluene.[6] Exposure to solvents such as toluene also increases your risk of miscarriage, and animal studies show that inhaling benzene vapors causes damaged reproductive organs and infertility.[7]

Toluene is a clear liquid that smells like paint thinner. It's added to gasoline to improve octane ratings. It's also used as a solvent in paints, coatings, synthetic fragrances, adhesives, inks and cleaning agents (particularly stain removers); and it's used in nail polish, glue, antifreeze and dyes. It's also in cigarette smoke.

Benzene is a very similar substance found in crude oil. It's a major component of gasoline, and is used in many of the same products as toluene (adhesives, cleaners, dyes, and so on) as well as pesticides, plastics, and synthetic fibers.

There are many ways you can get exposed to high levels of toluene, benzene, and other solvents. The simplest way is intentionally—people who huff paint, paint thinner, glue or similar substances to get high are inhaling very high levels of toluene. The second-simplest way is to work in an occupation where solvents are used regularly, for example: painter, printer, shoe manufacturer, hairdresser, nail technician, furniture finisher, rubber-plant worker and gas station worker.

And what if your significant other works in one of those fields? Well, that's a little more unclear. There have been studies that show differing results: Some say that male exposure to solvents didn't affect time to pregnancy when a couple was trying to conceive, but others say it did—and that men who are exposed to high levels of solvents have more abnormal and less motile sperm. Some studies found that low or moderate levels of exposure didn't pose a risk, but high levels had a profound effect.

What's clearer is that male exposure to high levels of solvents on the job is associated with higher rates of miscarriage, which does seem to back up the idea that the solvents cause more abnormal sperm.

## How to Avoid Toluene, Benzene and Other Solvents

1. If you can afford it, use full-service instead of self-service at the gas station and keep your window up except when needed so you don't breathe in fumes. If you have to pump your own, wash your hands afterwards.

2. When painting, keep windows open and choose paint with no or low VOCs, like Benjamin Moore's Natura line. Paint furniture outdoors.

3. Never use spray paint indoors. It's high in toluene and particularly bad for you because it's an aerosol-based spray that spreads tiny chemical particles through the air. Spray-on primers might look like tempting time-savers, but they're bad for your health.

4. Throughout your home use air purifiers that have VOC filters. Most air purifiers don't filter VOCs—you have to look for that designation specifically. Activated carbon filters are effective against VOCs. If you can afford to do it, have air purifiers running in every room of your house. If you can't, then at least use them in the bedrooms and the living room.

5. If you or your significant other work in a field where solvents are used, insist on proper ventilation. You need properly

maintained exhaust fans, open windows, air purifiers and any other precaution possible to keep the air quality in your workplace pure. When possible, work that involves VOCs should be taken outdoors.

6. Cheap dust masks do nothing to protect you from VOCs. You'll need a ventilator for that, which you can pick up at most home improvement stores or online for about $30.

7. Either don't wear nail polish, or pick nail polish without toluene. Google "toluene-free nail polish" for lists and reviews. When getting a manicure or pedicure, bring your own nail polish. Avoid gel manicures, which leave several layers of chemicals on your nails and require long acetone soaks to remove—while you're breathing in and soaking in a toxic chemical.

8. And while we're at it, "acetone-free" nail polish removers aren't all safe, either! You might assume so, based on their labels, but check what the acetone has been replaced by—in most cases, methanol or ethyl acetate. Methanol (also known as methyl alcohol) is another chemical solvent that is potentially even more dangerous than acetone. It's found in antifreeze, windshield wiper fluid, varnish, shellac, copy machine fluids and several other products, and high exposure to it can cause a laundry list of symptoms, such as seizures, nausea, vomiting, trouble breathing, blindness, blurred vision, convulsions, low blood pressure, comas, headaches, dizziness, pancreatitis, liver dysfunction, cramps and weakness. Fun stuff!

Ethyl acetate (also known as acetic ester, acetic ether, ethyl ester of acetic acid or ethyl ethanoate) is a flammable liquid used in a variety of products, including perfumes, cigarettes and glues. It's included in the list of hazardous chemicals from the National Institute for Occupational Safety and Health (NIOSH), and the NIOSH recommends no skin contact and use of a respirator when working with the chemical. It's known to be dangerous to the lungs, liver, kidney and heart, and it passes into breast milk. One study showed that 8 percent of lactating women's breast milk contained ethyl acetate.[8] This is considered one of the lesser-evil VOCs, and yet this is in the instructions given by the National Library of Medicine for advanced first aid for ethyl ethanoate exposure: "Consider orotracheal or nasotracheal intubation for airway control in the patient who is unconscious. Positive-pressure ventilation techniques with a bag-valve-mask device may be beneficial. Monitor cardiac rhythm and treat arrhythmias if necessary..."

These chemicals are not things you want in or on or around your body in any way, whether you're trying to get pregnant at the moment or not. But, in particular, you don't want them near you when there's any chance you could get pregnant because we know that they can pass to your baby as well. When you walk into a hair or nail salon and you can smell the chemicals strongly enough that your throat gets irritated, you have trouble breathing or your eyes water, *leave*. Always read labels. If you're going acetone-free, make sure the nail polish remover is water-based and free of all other solvents as well.

Understand that water-based nail polish removers aren't as effective, which means your nail polish isn't going to come off as easily. You're not just going to swipe it right off with a cotton ball; it's going to take some muscle and time. It's kind of a pain in the ass. But in the end, you won't have subjected yourself to a heap of toxic chemicals for the sake of having pretty nails.

# Keep Pesticides Out of Your Home

You know what cracks us up? When people buy organic food and then hire someone to come spray pesticides around their house. Certain pesticides have clearly been linked with both male and female fertility problems, and many other pesticides are suspected to have bad reproductive effects, though conclusive links have not yet been established. Both for your general health and for your fertility specifically, you want to stay away from pesticides and herbicides as much as you can.

The danger of pesticides is not just in eating them, but also in inhaling them. When you have pesticides on your lawn and garden and then you walk inside, you're tracking pesticides into your home. Even if it's not on your own property, anytime you walk around town, you're likely picking up pesticides and other chemicals on your shoes. Make it a habit to take off your shoes indoors and either just wear socks or slippers, or have a separate pair of "indoor shoes."

And before you turn to conventional pesticides if you have a pest problem, consider that there may be safer options that are just as effective. For example, food-grade diatomaceous earth is a bug killer that you can actually eat! It's a white powdery substance made from the fossilized remains of a type of algae. It contains mostly silica, and you sprinkle it around your home (inside and out) using a bellows duster to help get rid of any kinds of bugs with exoskeletons—such as bedbugs, roaches, ants, fleas, pillbugs and crickets.

Boric acid is another nontoxic pest control agent for crawling insects, and bait boxes for rodents are safer than pellets and powders. Cornmeal kills ants, citrus peels around the garden deter many types of bugs and cedar deters moths.

We know that you may not have a choice about pesticide usage if you live in an apartment complex, dorm or other group housing situation. If you have the ability to ask before you move in, find out what the pest management plan is for the building before making your decision. You may find that some buildings are better than others in terms of doing inspections and getting to the root of problems, rather than just reflexively spraying the building every few months.

"When I lived in a condo complex, the homeowners' board sent out a flyer warning us to keep our pets indoors on Friday because the maintenance company was going to spray pesticides," says expectant mother Anna. "I wasn't sure if I really had a choice in the matter, but I called the office and asked them not to spray my property. They obliged. Of course, all of the neighboring properties were still sprayed, so it's not like I was able to eliminate it from my environment entirely, but I like to think that every little bit helps."

# Fighting Formaldehyde

Ahh, formaldehyde ... that chemical best known for embalming dead people. (Or, in the case of biology class, frogs ready for dissection.) But did you know that formaldehyde is also used to make cabinets (nearly all kitchen cabinets contain some level of added formaldehyde), furniture, cigarettes, wrinkle-resistant fabrics, car parts, disinfectants and many cosmetics, and it's emitted by kerosene space heaters and gas stoves?

It irritates the airways and is known to cause cancer and reproductive problems, and if ingested or inhaled in large doses, death. The Occupational Safety and Health Administration (OSHA) takes formaldehyde exposure in the workplace seriously and requires companies to take reasonable measures to protect their workers from exposure.

But just as we see when industries want to protect their use of other dangerous chemicals, the cabinet- and furniture-making industries are trying very hard to make us think that formaldehyde is an awesome gift to our lives. A video on www.greencabinetsource.com that tries to make formaldehyde sound fun has the narrator saying this: "Sitting right here on the vanity, these everyday cosmetics also benefit from formaldehyde, which inhibits the growth of bacteria and preserves the product. Without it, shampoo wouldn't be germ-free and other products wouldn't last nearly as long." In another such video, the narrator smiles a Pleasantville sort of smile while holding a mug of coffee and informing us happily that her coffee contains formaldehyde, too. And it's totally fine!

Jeez, Louise. What a load.

Cosmetics don't benefit from formaldehyde. And your shampoo doesn't need to be laced with poison to be "germ-free." There are plenty of shampoos without any formaldehyde and no one seems to be catching the plague from them.

It is true that there is some formaldehyde naturally occurring in wood. You can't help that. But cabinet and furniture makers don't need to add extra formaldehyde. Most of them do, but there are alternatives. And among those that do, there's a wide range of how much formaldehyde they use.

As far as fertility goes, there have been numerous conflicting studies trying to determine whether or not formaldehyde has reproductive system effects. Researchers in a recent review concluded that the chemical mostly affects the respiratory system and is broken down by the time it would reach the reproductive organs, and yet there is evidence that miscarriage rates go up when either the woman or the man in a couple have ongoing exposure to formaldehyde. It's one of the "big, bad" chemicals that's actually classified as a known carcinogen (it takes a lot to get to that label—it's not a "possible" or "probable" carcinogen), so I wouldn't wait until the evidence about fertility is absolutely conclusive. It's something to avoid as much as possible if you want to be healthy enough to play with those future kids of yours, at the very least.

# Brazilian Blowouts and Keratin Treatments

Hear us on this: Don't get a Brazilian Blowout or other keratin treatment without *absolutely knowing* what's in it.

When the hair-straightening and smoothing process known as Brazilian Blowouts became really popular a few years back, concerned people investigated and discovered that there was a lot of formaldehyde in these treatments. Word got out, the Brazilian Blowout people had a PR problem, and they responded by swearing up and down that their treatments did not contain formaldehyde and were totally safe. In fact, their website said this:

> **"The ONLY Professional Smoothing Treatment that improves the health of the hair. No Damage! and No harsh chemicals! CONTAINS NO FORMALDEHYDE!!"**

That was a lie. A grammatically screwed-up lie. It hurts our brains just to copy it into our book.

Formaldehyde wasn't directly added to the ingredients, but it did contain ingredients that emitted formaldehyde into the air while the product was being applied, and left formaldehyde in the hair afterwards, too—which the company knew. One of its ingredients is methylene glycol, and you know what that is? Formaldehyde with water added to it so it becomes a technically different chemical.

Stylists had been complaining about nosebleeds, respiratory problems (including chronic bronchitis, pneumonia and wheezing), eye irritation, dry and sore throats, chest pain, loss of sense of smell, dizziness and many other symptoms consistent with chemical poisoning. Customers had run to their doctors with ongoing health problems related to their hair treatment.

After two lawsuits (for which the company paid abour $4.2 million in damages), their products now need to bear a brightly colored and clear warning sticker that states they contain methylene glycol, which emits formaldehyde during the heating process, and that the product should be applied only in a well-ventilated space.

Brazilian Blowout took most of the bad press, but they are far from the only company of their kind—lots of the "keratin treatments" or "keratin blowouts" or "straightening treatments" offered at salons also contain formaldehyde and other dangerous chemicals. You wouldn't necessarily know that from the ingredients lists, though—you'll rarely see formaldehyde there. OSHA has put out a fact sheet detailing the results of its investigation into these hair-straightening treatments: OSHA cited several salons and beauty schools for having too-high levels of formaldehyde in the air, failing to protect their workers, failing to educate their workers about safety precautions and otherwise failing to follow the agency's guidelines about formaldehyde safety. The report also found that many products had deceptive advertising or ingredients lists, claiming to be formaldehyde-free when they weren't.[9]

OSHA lists the following as synonyms for *formaldehyde* or *chemicals that release formaldehyde*: methylene glycol, formalin, methylene oxide, paraform, formic aldehyde, methanal, oxomethane, oxymethylene, timonacic acid and thiazolidinecarboxylic acid.

Luckily, you don't have to worry as much about keratin shampoos, conditioners and styling products. OSHA found that they contained far less formaldehyde—to put it in perspective, all the samples contained between .01 and .05 percent formaldehyde, whereas Brazilian

Blowout Acai Solution contained 8.8 percent formaldehyde. You still don't want any formaldehyde, but don't get too nervous if you've already used the over-the-counter products as opposed to the chemical process in the salon.

Check the Resources section at the back of the book for a list of brands to avoid.

## How to Avoid Formaldehyde in Other Stuff

- If you're getting new kitchen cabinets, opt for all real wood, not particle board or pressed wood. Particle board and pressed wood require more glue, which typically contains more formaldehyde. Even though we just made fun of www.greencabinetsource.com for its silly pro-formaldehyde videos, this site is a good source to check for manufacturers that adhere to the industry's strictest emissions standards.

- Medium density fiberboard (MDF) is the absolute worst. Avoid it.

- Formaldehyde emissions significantly go down over time in cabinets and furniture. If you can buy good-quality used cabinets and furniture, rather than new, you'll most likely have lower formaldehyde levels in your home.

- There are two types of formaldehydes in cosmetics. It may be added directly, or chemicals that give off formaldehyde may be used. The four most common formaldehyde-emitting chemicals to watch out for on an ingredients list are quaternium-15, diazolidinyl urea, imidazolidinly urea and DMDM hydantoin.

- If possible, get your hair done at home or during a time of day when the salon isn't busy, to limit your exposure to the chemicals used there.

- If you have a fireplace, make sure to have your chimney cleaned every year and keep it free of obstructions. The more smoke that gets into your home, the more formaldehyde.

- Don't let anyone smoke in your home.

- Close windows and doors when you're using lawn mowers, leaf blowers, and other gas-powered tools outside. You don't want those fumes in your house.

- Use air purifiers in your home that contain VOC filters.

# Oh, FML, Just Tell Me Where to Find Safe Products

It's not always easy to find the safest products in big department stores. If they're even there, it requires a lot of label-reading and reading between the lines to get to what you're looking for. Here are some shortcuts:

- **WWW.EWG.ORG/SKINDEEP:** This is an amazing list of cosmetics, sunscreens, body lotions, deodorants and other health and beauty products, all identified with descriptions of their ingredients and a safety rating from 0 to 10 (low hazard to high hazard). It's run by the Environmental Working Group, a nonprofit organization that got tired of the fact that our government doesn't require testing of the chemicals used in personal care products and set out to educate people about what we're using on our bodies. In doing so, they've already reformed the sunscreen industry—when they started, they did such a good job of exposing unsafe ingredients in most sunscreens that they essentially forced sunscreen companies to make better products or risk losing too much market share.

- **WWW.THESOFTLANDING.COM:** Three sisters and their mom started this company in 2007 in response to the frequent recalls and scares about BPA and other chemicals in baby products. While their original focus was on baby products, they've expanded to include many other products that you might be concerned about in a home, from food dehydrators to coffeemakers. What's nice is that they also have a few "shopping guides" that point out product categories you might not even have thought about when it comes to finding safer alternatives.

- **WWW.GOODGUIDE.COM:** Led by a team of scientists and professors at UC Berkeley, this one is similar in style to the Environmental Working Group's Skin Deep database, but a lot more comprehensive—it not only covers personal care products, but also food, electronics, clothing, pet food and more. It ranks everything on a 1–10 scale according to health properties as well as the company's environmental and social policies. That can make things a little confusing because you have to look into the reasoning behind each score before assuming that a low-scoring product is unsafe. For example, several crystal deodorant stones rate only between 5 and 6, even though there are no known health concerns. The ratings may be lowered based on things like a company's record of diversity in the workplace or the lack of recyclable packaging. But the ratings are also broken down into the three categories on each product's individual page, so you don't have to look too far.

# NASA's List of Awesome House Plants

A NASA scientist, Bill Wolverton, was tasked with improving the air quality in space shuttles on outer space missions, and he wanted to see if houseplants would clean the air and absorb nasty chemicals. It turned out that some were better at it than others. Of course, he knew that his findings would also apply to people who still had their feet firmly on planet Earth. Wolverton explained that the plants mostly help in energy-efficient, nonventilated buildings. In houses with good ventilation, air exchange moves quickly enough that the plants' air-cleaning value is not as important. Based on Wolverton's work, researcher Luz Claudio came up with a top 10 list of best air-cleaning houseplants, judged by how well they remove chemical vapors, how easy they are to maintain, how prone they are to insect infestation and how quickly they transpire water. Might want to keep these around your home or office, particularly if your ventilation is not so hot.

1. Areca palm
2. Lady palm
3. Bamboo palm
4. Rubber plant
5. Dracaena
6. English ivy
7. Dwarf date palm
8. Ficus
9. Boston fern
10. Peace lily

Remember to care for your houseplants properly, though—too much water in the soil or sitting on the leaves and they'll develop mold, which is also harmful for your health.

## Final Thoughts

Look, here's what we're saying: Before Kyra started trying to have a baby, she didn't know a phthalate from a potato. She didn't care enough about her own health until she realized it could have an effect on someone else's health: a totally innocent newborn baby. And, yes, it's a pain in the butt to have to research and figure out which products have these sorts of chemicals and which don't, and you can make yourself crazy in the process if you try to avoid them all the time. You can't. It's not possible. You can only minimize your exposure to them, speak up in the fight for labeling and better safety measures in manufacturing, and then let go—no use worrying about things that are out of your control.

# Chapter 7
# Eat, Drink and Be Fertile

Let's talk about digestion and nutrition: They play a key role in just about every aspect of our health, including fertility. What you eat and drink affect the way your body works for better or worse—so let's make sure you understand how to properly nourish yourself.

## Your Lovely Liver

Livers are pretty amazing workaholics that rarely get the credit they deserve. Your liver is the largest organ in your body, aside from your skin. It's kind of triangular-shaped and weighs about three pounds. It's in your abdomen, mostly on the right side of your stomach, but you can't feel it because it's protected by your rib cage. It's essentially in charge of processing everything that goes into your body—whether you eat it, drink it, inhale it or absorb it through your skin, it has to go through the liver, where all that stuff gets filtered and either thrown out, redirected, stored or converted into something useful.

Livers get their proper credit mostly when we're talking about alcoholism. You probably know that alcoholics have to worry about things like cirrhosis of the liver (permanent scarring that makes it difficult for the liver to function) because they overburden their livers so much. But did you know why they get overburdened? They're multitasking like crazy, doing all these things at once:

1. Making bile to break down fats and clean up your blood to prevent jaundice. Bile carries your waste to your intestine so it can be turned into poop.

2. Breaking down nutrients into usable stuff (like glucose and ATP) for distribution all over your body.

3. Making proteins, including some that act as hormone transporters.

4. Storing vitamins and minerals, particularly iron.

5. Storing glycogen, then converting it into glucose and releasing it when your body needs some backup fuel.

6. Detoxing your body, not only from things like alcohol and illegal drugs but also from prescription drugs, crappy chemicals added to processed foods, pesticides sprayed on your fruit, heavy oils, and so on.

7. Getting rid of old, worn-out red blood cells.

8. Helping with blood clotting.

9. Making cholesterol (not always a bad thing—you need some cholesterol to live).

10. Functioning as part of your immune system.

11. Regulating your sex hormone levels and getting rid of excess hormones.

That last one is a big component of fertility, as you might guess, so let's discuss how this works.

For your body to run the way it's meant to, you need a certain balance of hormones. Women in their childbearing years need to have fairly high levels of estrogen for the first half of their cycle before ovulation each month, and then progesterone balances out the estrogen after ovulation.

You don't want to have too little estrogen or you may experience the symptoms of menopause, such as a lack of ovulation, infertility, a slower metabolism, growth of facial hair, vaginal dryness, hot flashes, night sweats, fatigue, mood changes, thinning hair, decreased sex drive, osteoporosis (bone loss), memory loss, osteoarthritis, digestive problems, bloating, irritability . . . yeah, I'd be irritable, too, if I were going through all that stuff. Aren't you looking forward to menopause now?

The huge drop in estrogen after childbirth is also most likely to blame for postpartum depression and its lesser counterpart, the "baby blues."

Now, the funny(ish) thing is that some of the symptoms that accompany lack of estrogen are the same as the symptoms that accompany too much estrogen, or "estrogen dominance." Hormones are weird little things that don't neatly line up into categories. There's still a lot of mystery surrounding exactly how they affect us and how we can effectively keep them in balance. But if you have too much estrogen in relation to your progesterone levels, you might have to deal with ovarian cysts, weight gain, fibrocystic breast disease, migraines, heavy or irregular menstrual periods, endometriosis, weight gain and breast cancer. You can get a blood test to determine if you're estrogen-dominant or estrogen-deficient.

For fertility to work right, your hormones need to work right—and part of what determines if your hormones are "working right" is your liver function.

Your liver needs to be able to filter out any excess hormones, and it's good at doing that, unless it gets overworked. Picture a secretary whose job it is to type up reports, file them and send out mail. Now picture that her workload suddenly triples and she has to find a way to keep up. What's going to happen? She's going to get sloppy. Some things are going to fall through the cracks, get misfiled or fall off the desk.

So it is with your liver. When it gets backed up, things go wrong. Normally, any extra estrogen is carried out of the liver by the bile, taken for a trip through your intestines and then excreted or reabsorbed. But if your liver gets backed up, then the extra estrogen just stays in your bloodstream, like a party guest who won't leave at the end of the night.

Sometimes you can't help it—your liver may be overtaxed because of factors beyond your control, or it might be overtaxed because of things you're consuming. For instance...

## Fatty Foods

You need to have some dietary fat to stay alive, but as I'm sure you've noticed, most Americans are not in danger of eating too little fat. We're in the midst of an obesity epidemic that has led to, among other things, a huge increase in Nonalcoholic Fatty Liver Disease (NFLD), the name of the condition when the content of the liver is more than 5–10 percent fat. It's directly correlated with obesity—the more obese the person is, the higher the risk of NFLD.

You want to choose healthy fats for your diet—monounsaturated and polyunsaturated fats. As much as possible, avoid saturated fats and especially trans fats, as both raise your "bad" cholesterol level. Saturated fats mostly come from animal food sources (meat and dairy) and trans fats mostly come from processed foods, when oils are combined with hydrogen to make them stay solid at room temperature. That makes them more shelf-stable and easier to cook with, but it also makes them totally unhealthy. If you see the words "partially hydrogenated" oil on the label, don't put it into your grocery cart.

You can also easily get caught in the "low-fat" and "fat-free" trap. Low-fat/fat-free doesn't always mean healthy! In fact, lots of times, a manufacturer adds in heaps of other unhealthy stuff for flavoring to make up for the lack of fat, so you wind up getting a fat-free mouthful of sugar, artificial sweeteners and other junk that's potentially worse for you than the fat was in the first place.

| GOOD FATS | BAD FATS |
|---|---|
| Plant-based oils such as olive, sunflower, peanut, corn, safflower, and canola oil (in moderation) | Butter and margarine |
| Avocado | Red meat |
| Nuts | Heavy cream |
| Fish | Pizza, bagels, pastries |
| Olives | Fried food |
| Seeds | Candy bars |

## Sugar

Speaking of sugar, that's a major contributing factor to overtaxing your liver. Type 2 diabetes is being diagnosed at record rates, and it's often the result of overloading your body with sugar until your liver and pancreas can't keep up and then go haywire.

Now is a good time to give up your soft-drink habit. It's like drinking a bag of sugar. As with any other habit, it can be difficult to change your routine and give up your beloved Dr. Pepper or Coke. But you know what's amazing? After about six months off the stuff, you probably won't even like the taste anymore. You'll wonder how you ever drank such sickeningly sweet garbage in the first place. Hard to believe now, we know, but your tastes actually do change. It can take a while to acquire a taste for healthful foods and drink, but once you break that sugar cycle, you won't miss it the way you think you will.

It can be very confusing to spot sugar on an ingredients label. But if you see any of these things, every one of them means "sugar."

- anhydrous dextrose
- corn syrup
- crystal dextrose
- evaporated corn sweetener
- fruit juice concentrate
- glucose
- honey
- liquid fructose
- malt syrup
- maple syrup
- pancake syrup
- cane juice
- corn syrup solids
- dextrose
- fructose
- fruit nectar
- high-fructose corn syrup (HFCS)
- lactose
- maltose
- molasses
- sucrose

Then there are the artificial sweeteners and sugar alcohols, which also tax the liver:

- Acesulfame potassium
- Erythritol
- Isomalt
- Maltitol
- Neotame
- Sorbitol
- Xylitol
- Aspartame
- Hydrogenated starch hydrolysate
- Lactitol
- Mannitol
- Saccharine
- Sucralose

## Crash Diets

If you are overweight, of course it's a great idea to lose weight—but dropping pounds too quickly can damage your liver and is a risk factor in NFLD. Losing weight too quickly also makes your body think it's starving, which slows down your metabolism because your body thinks it had better hang on to everything you eat. That makes it so much easier to put weight back on if you stop dieting or slip up, and you'll typically gain back more weight than you lost, which is what starts the cycle of yo-yo dieting. As you can imagine, your body hates yo-yo dieting. It has no idea what the heck you're doing to it.

## Nonorganic Fruits and Vegetables

Fruits and vegetables are wonderful for your fertility, but the pesticides that come along with nonorganic produce are not. Your liver has to get rid of all those pesticides, which adds to its normal burden. We know that it can be difficult to eat a wholly organic diet because of the expense and because organic foods are not always readily available. But some foods are more important than others when you're deciding between organic and nonorganic. In general, fruits and vegetables that have thick skins are less likely to be laden with pesticides and fungicides.

The Environmental Working Group (EWG) puts out a list of the "Dirty Dozen Plus" (twelve fruits and vegetables most likely to contain pesticide residues, plus two that contain exceptionally toxic pesticides) and the "Clean Fifteen" (those least likely to contain pesticide residues). EWG researchers update that list annually, based on their most recent testing. They base their lists on U.S. Department of Agriculture (USDA) and FDA testing, where they wash and peel produce that's meant to be eaten that way and then they check it for multiple types of pesticides. Almost 70 percent of conventionally grown produce tests positive for pesticide residue after washing or peeling, meaning that no matter how well you wash your strawberries or lettuce, you're most likely eating pesticides unless you're buying organic.

Unfortunately, one of the former "Clean Fifteen" honorees—bananas—dropped off the list in a big way in 2013, so it's important to check in annually and see if anything has changed. If you can't afford to buy everything organic, here are the two current cheat sheets. Everything's listed in alphabetical order, not ranked from best to worse or vice versa:

| DIRTY DOZEN | CLEAN FIFTEEN |
|---|---|
| Apples | Asparagus |
| Celery | Avocados |
| Cherry tomatoes | Cabbage |
| Cucumbers | Cantaloupe |
| Grapes | Sweet corn |
| Hot peppers | Eggplant |
| Nectarines (imported) | Grapefruit |
| Peaches | Kiwi |
| Potatoes | Mangoes |
| Spinach | Mushrooms |
| Strawberries | Onions |
| Sweet bell peppers | Papayas |
| **PLUS** | Sweet peas |
| Contaminated with pesticides that are being phased out of agriculture because they're particularly toxic: | Pineapples |
| | Sweet potatoes |
| Kale/collard greens | |
| Squash (domestic) | |

If you have room in your yard, why not grow your own organic garden this summer? You can freeze, can or dehydrate your harvest to save for the cooler months as well. Using a home dehydrator is better than buying commercially dried fruits and vegetables, which lose more nutrients and often contain added sweeteners that can overtax your liver.

Think of the time spent in your garden as a gift to your fertility in multiple ways: You're providing clean and healthy produce for your body, getting exercise and vitamin D—both of which are good for fertility—and it can be a form of stress management. And if you keep it up, one day you can mash up those organic fruits and veggies for your future baby.

## Nonorganic Dairy and Meat

Dairy products are one of the most important categories to buy organic. Milk that's not organic often has added recombinant bovine growth hormone (rBGH), meant to make the cows produce more milk. It's a genetically engineered hormone that originally gets injected into a cow and tricks her body into thinking she just had a calf and needs to provide for it (so she produces more milk). It comes with some serious drawbacks for both the cow and us—for one thing, it seriously increases the cow's risk of mastitis. Mastitis is the infection and inflammation of the mammary gland and udder. It can make the cow sick, and it can make the milk watery or chunky and tainted with pus and bacteria. To treat it, dairy farmers typically inject the infected cows with antibiotics and steroids.

The engineered hormone is sold under the trade name POSILAC, and the FDA requires it to be sold with an insert warning of its known dangers, including reduced pregnancy rates, increased risk for mastitis, increased risk of subclinical mastitis (milk not visibly abnormal), more therapeutic drug treatment for mastitis and other health problems, and enlarged hocks and disorders of the foot region.

Not sure about you, but milk that's teeming with pus and antibiotics to treat infections sounds *delicious* to us!

On an organic farm, cows are given organic feed and can't be fed genetically modified foods or given growth hormones.

Neither system is perfect; even on organic farms, cows can be fed some pretty gross stuff, including "poultry waste" (aka chicken droppings), but at least you have a much better chance of drinking what you expect—milk—rather than a glass full of unexpected chemicals. You also have a better chance that the animals are treated humanely.

## Meat

Meat is another important food group to eat organically. Livestock on conventional farms (aka feedlots) are frequently given growth hormones and antibiotics to prevent disease. It's not yet possible to say what all those added hormones are doing to our bodies or our children's bodies. There are lots of theories that these types of added hormones are what's causing the surge of early puberty. Menstrual periods are still starting at about the same time, but whereas the average age for the onset of puberty (the development of breasts) has always been between eleven and twelve, it is now eight or nine—eight for African-American girls and nine for Caucasian girls. And there are more and more cases of what doctors call "precocious puberty"—girls who develop way before normal, like a girl who started growing pubic hair at age four, and another with pimples and underarm odor at three. To add insult to injury, precocious puberty is also associated with breast cancer down the line.

Are these effects of nonorganic meat? Possibly. No one can make the direct link yet, because there are so many other factors and possibilities in our everyday lives. But if it's not specifically the meat, it certainly may be the buildup of the many products and foods that have estrogenic effects—things that weren't around fifty years ago.

There are two reasons not to eat nonorganic dairy and meat with regard to your fertility: First, you don't know what effect all those extra hormones and antibiotics will have on you or your future children (but it's unlikely to be a fun effect), and second, your liver hates this stuff. It just wants to do its job in peace and not have to deal with having to filter out more unnatural garbage.

---

### Natural versus Organic

Natural is not the same as organic. Actually, natural means nothing because there's no regulation about how the word needs to be used on product packaging. Products with genetically modified organisms (GMOs) and artificial sweeteners have used the "natural" label. However, the USDA Organic seal means that a product is at least 95 percent organic and that the fields and processing facilities for these products have been inspected and periodically tested to make sure they're following protocol, which includes not administering routine antibiotics and growth hormones, not using artificial sweeteners or coloring, and avoiding most preservatives. Soil and water samples are checked periodically as well, testing for pesticides and fertilizers that would go against regulations.

---

## Alcohol

Alcohol puts stress on your liver whether you abuse it or not. Obviously, it's worse if you binge-drink or drink every day, but even moderate alcohol use can be tough for your liver to process, particularly if it's overworked by other things. Kim Ross, holistic nutritionist for the NYU Fertility Center, recommends that when you reach the point where you want to get pregnant soon, you should limit yourself to about three drinks a week—red wine, preferably, because it contains the phytonutrient resveratrol, which has antioxidant and anti-inflammatory properties and can help prevent insulin resistance.

# What to Eat for Better Fertility

Aside from the things to avoid, there are also things you should eat in order to retain or improve your fertility.

### Whole grains, such as beans, brown rice and unrefined breads:

Refined carbs (white bread, white rice, sugar) cause an increase in blood sugar and insulin in the body that can disrupt hormones and your ovulation cycle, but whole grains don't have this effect.

### Lean meats:

Iron is an important nutrient to aid fertility, and the easiest way to get iron in your diet is through meat—but it should be lean meat. Choose lean cuts; trim the fat; and bake, grill or broil instead of frying. Studies show that women who increase their iron intake during the preconception period have a higher fertility rate than women who are iron-deficient. Just don't overdo your consumption of meat because it can decrease fertility. If you're a vegan, you may need to take a vitamin with iron in it.

### Omega-3 fish:

Salmon, sardines, herring and other types of fatty fish boost fertility, thanks to their high levels of omega-3 fatty acids. Not only will they increase blood flow to reproductive organs, but they also regulate reproductive hormones. Vegans will benefit from omega-3 fatty acids from flaxseed, almonds, walnuts, pumpkin seeds and DHA-enriched eggs.

### Organic dairy:

Milk, cheese, yogurt and other dairy sources are good for bone health as well as reproductive health. Some research shows women who have problems with ovulation may benefit from splurging on a serving a day of full-fat dairy.

### Organic raspberries and blueberries:

All fruits and vegetables are great for you, but these berries are particularly good for fertility. Packed with antioxidants, they protect your body from cell damage and cell aging—and this includes cells in your reproductive system and your eggs.

### Healthy fats, such as canola oil, olive oil, flaxseed oil, nuts and avocados:

Kim Ross suggests consuming as many high-water-content, nutrient-dense foods as possible—whole foods from the earth. When she counsels fertility clients, she advises them to go with an 80 percent plant-based diet along the lines of the Mediterranean diet because it's anti-aging and decreases chances of disease—anything from polycystic ovarian syndrome (PCOS) to cancer.

"You really can get adequate protein from a mostly vegetarian diet," she says. "It's the best way to get the vitamins, minerals and fiber you need."

You can learn about the Mediterranean diet online or in a number of books (such as *The Mediterranean Prescription* by Angelo Aquista,

MD or *The Mediterranean Diet Cookbook* by Rockridge Press). Among the main tenets of the Mediterranean diet are:

- Eat lots of fresh fruits and vegetables that are in season.
- Stick to small amounts of red meat—just two to three times a month.
- Eat fish and poultry at least twice a week.
- Replace butter and margarine with olive oil or other healthy fats.
- Choose a variety of whole grains (barley, oats, buckwheat, rye and so on).
- Eat a daily serving of nuts.

This type of diet improves your overall health, which includes your reproductive health.

## Fill Up on Fiber

Fiber is another tool to flush out excess estrogen, says Kim Ross. Fiber adds bulk to your digestion and helps you feel full. It also helps prevent constipation, which keeps things "moving right along." When you have a diet with inadequate fiber, you can slow down your digestive system and the estrogen that's sitting in your bowel waiting to make its exit can get bored waiting and get reabsorbed into your system, causing a buildup of too much estrogen.

Now here's the thing about adding fiber to your diet: Do it slowly. I'm just sayin'. There's this friend we have who realized she needed to add fiber to her diet, promptly launched into a day filled with salad, a Fiber One bar and high-fiber bread, and basically didn't come out of the bathroom the whole next day. Your body needs time to adjust. Otherwise, it's thinking, "GET ALL THIS STUFF OUT

IMMEDIATELY!" Fiber causes gas, bloating, diarrhea and stomach cramps when you consume too much too fast.

Pay attention to ingredients labels: You want to aim for about 25 grams a day (that's the recommended daily intake level for women; men should get 38 grams), whereas most American women get about half that amount per day. If you're not getting enough, then build up to optimal levels slowly over the course of about three weeks. You can use dietary supplements, but it's better to get your fiber from food for several reasons—one of which is that foods that are high in fiber are typically very good for you all around (such as fruits and vegetables that also contain important vitamins), and you can control the intake of fiber gradually throughout the day, rather than taking just one big dose.

## Good Sources of Fiber

Fruits: raspberries, prunes, raisins, pears, blackberries, apples

Legumes: navy beans, black beans, split peas, pinto beans, kidney beans, lentils, lima beans

Other vegetables: artichokes, green peas, broccoli, Brussels sprouts, sweet corn

Grains, pasta and cereal: whole-wheat spaghetti, rye bread, whole-wheat bread, bran flakes, oat-bran muffins

Nuts and seeds: sunflower seeds, pistachios, almonds, pecans, walnuts, peanuts

# Probiotics

If you have a sensitive stomach, you may want to limit your dairy intake, which is hard for many people to digest even without a clinical lactose intolerance. But Kim Ross makes an exception for yogurt because it contains probiotics—which have the opposite effect. Probiotics are great for your gut, and, like fiber, they can help your digestive system work better and improve your immune function, which improves your fertility as well.

You can take a daily probiotic supplement, such as Acidophilus Pearls or Accuflora (available at drugstores), or you can get probiotics from your diet. Good sources, aside from yogurt, include kefir, sauerkraut and miso.

## Watch Out for Mercury

Mercury is a toxic metal that exists naturally in the environment, and is released into the air and water through industrial pollution. Fish are contaminated with mercury when they swim in polluted water; some fish retain mercury more than others, with a general rule being that the bigger and older the fish, the higher the mercury content. Mercury is also used in amalgam dental fillings and as a preservative in vaccines.

Starting in 1991, the World Health Organization stated that when it comes to mercury, "The exposure of women in childbearing age should be as low as possible." That's because mercury exposure has been linked to infertility, miscarriage and a host of birth defects and neurological problems. That doesn't mean that you should avoid fish—quite the opposite—fish and shellfish are great sources of protein and omega-3s and are low in fat, so you should include fish in your diet about twice a week. However, you should stick to fish known to be low in mercury.

continued on page 138

"Even one serving of tuna is too much," says Kim Ross. Albacore (white) tuna has more mercury than canned light tuna.

The FDA suggests that women of childbearing age and children completely avoid shark, swordfish, king mackerel and tilefish, which rank the highest in mercury content. Among the lowest in mercury are:

- Shrimp
- Salmon
- Pollock
- Catfish

Fish sticks and fish patties for sandwiches are typically made with cod, haddock or pollock, with some premium types made with tilapia. All those types of fish are low in mercury.

Call your local health department to find out about fish that you or someone you know has caught locally; you may find out that there are warnings about higher-than-average mercury levels in certain types of fish caught in your area.

# Detox Diets

When she counsels patients, Kim Ross comes up with a personalized diet and detox plan based on their health background so that they can start with a clean environment working optimally. She says that detox plan is particularly important for people with digestive trouble.

"If you have an inflamed digestive tract because of a health problem, such as irritable bowel syndrome, Crohn's, colitis, PCOS or type 2 diabetes, a short-term detox for two weeks can really improve your digestive function, relax your body and decrease inflammation. And then more energy can go toward your reproductive system," says Kim.

When your body is not functioning right, it's wasting energy on dealing with the problems and stealing energy from your other systems—that's why, for example, you may feel extra-tired and lose your appetite when you have a cold. Your body is spending its limited energy fighting off the illness, shunting energy away from other bodily functions, like digestion and creative thinking. So it is with fertility: The more you can solve your health problems and get your body working at its peak, the more your reproductive system can work at its best, too.

Detox diets typically consist of lots of fresh fruits, vegetables and water, and lack any processed foods, dairy, wheat, caffeine and fried foods. Check with your doctor before starting a detox plan to make sure you're in good enough health—people with liver or kidney problems shouldn't do it, and women who are pregnant or nursing shouldn't, either. There can be serious gastrointestinal side effects from all the extra fiber, so you might want to start on a weekend or days off work or school.

Kim also mentions that when you're actually trying to get pregnant, you shouldn't drink anything ice cold—room temperature drinks are much easier on the digestive tract, again making things more efficient so that energy can be conserved for the reproductive organs.

# PFOA, PTFE, PFOS, and the Question of Cookware

You may have noticed the growing market for "green" cookware—pots and pans that either don't have nonstick properties or advertise themselves as PFOA- and PTFE-free.

Nonstick is pretty awesome—who wants to use elbow grease to scrub sauce and breading out of a pan when you could just give it a quick rinse instead? We Americans are not known for our desire to make life harder on ourselves, so when Teflon came onto the market, it was a very big deal. In the 1940s, it was used for industrial purposes, but in 1961, the first Teflon-coated frying pan was marketed in the United States. Suddenly you could cook scrambled eggs and not have to spend the next ten minutes scraping the residue off the pan.

Teflon is a brand name of the human-made chemical polytetrafluoroethylene (PTFE), known as the most "slippery substance" in existence. It's attached to pots and pans by another human-made chemical called perfluorooctanoic acid (PFOA). Most of the PFOA is burned off in the manufacturing process.

Pots and pans aren't the only places you'll find these chemicals in the kitchen. They may also line your oven or your stove's drip pans, making it easier to clean them as well.

However, there has been ongoing controversy about the safety of these two chemicals.

First, the one thing that's been proven: Birds die if they're around nonstick cookware that's overheated, or a nonstick-coated oven that's set too high (such as on the self-cleaning cycle—which really just uses extremely high heat to burn off residue). The nonstick surface gives off fumes that are toxic to birds and can kill them within about a minute. If you have pet birds, either you shouldn't use nonstick cookware at all or you should keep the birds far away from the kitchen.

But as far as the other stuff goes, it's a lot less clear.

We can probably set aside the rumors about flaking Teflon. While it's not appetizing to see pieces of Teflon in your stir-fry, it also hasn't been found to be dangerous. Eating flakes of this chemical isn't a big deal; inhaling the fumes from the PFOA may be.

We know that when Teflon-coated cookware is heated at very high temperatures, people can get something known as "Teflon flu," or "Polymer fume fever." That's when you get flulike symptoms temporarily from inhaling the fumes. But as far as long-term exposure to this cookware at normal-ish temperatures, it's questionable. We know that this chemical can stay in our bodies for a long time and it isn't easily broken down. We also know that it's present in the environment and in most people's bloodstreams at low levels. And we know that studies on lab animals have shown it to have detrimental effects on their development.

Because of this, the Environmental Protection Agency (EPA) began investigating PFOA in the 1990s, eventually taking action against DuPont (makers of Teflon) for "multiple failures to report information to the EPA about substantial risk of injury to human health or the environment from PFOA." DuPont settled the case for $10.25 million, the largest civil administrative penalty the EPA has ever collected. They've also imposed a plan for PFOA to be entirely phased out of new cookware starting in 2015.

Even considering that, however, human studies of PTFE and PFOA are inconclusive.

If you heat your Teflon over 500°F (which is mostly a problem if you forget something on the stove, if you preheat a dry pan too long or if you use the self-clean function on your oven), it releases a whole cacophony of toxic chemicals into the air. But if you use it at normal temperatures, even when it's scratched, it doesn't appear to cause health problems.

To complicate the issue, however, PFOA (and a similar human-made chemical, PFOS) is not just found in cookware, but also in carpets, fabrics, food packaging, insecticides and many other household products—so it's hard to study the effect of what's in your cookware only, because you're likely exposed to the chemicals multiple times per day outside of the kitchen.

And here's where it all gets fuzzy in terms of fertility: In 2009, researchers from UCLA published the results of their research on

1,240 pregnant Danish women. In the study, the women were asked how long it took them to get pregnant, and their blood was tested for PFOA and PFOS. Then, according to how high the levels of chemicals were, the women were categorized into four groups. The women with the lowest levels of these chemicals were considered the reference group. Those in the other three groups were found to be twice as likely to have taken at least a year to get pregnant, or to need infertility treatments, as compared to the reference group.[1]

So where did the chemicals come from that wound up in their bloodstream? It could have been any number of places, but cookware was not likely a significant source of it. Since most PFOA is burned off during the manufacturing process, it's more likely that it's simply become an environmental contaminant now.

There have also been several studies to figure out if high levels of PFOA and PFOS exposure lead to miscarriage, birth defects and problems within pregnancy, again with inconclusive results.

So we don't think you need to run out and toss your Teflon, as long as you're not in the habit of forgetting it on the stove and letting it overheat. But it's up to you what to do with this information: If you want to cross this concern completely off your list and it'll help you feel better, then buy either stainless-steel or cast-iron cookware. Cast iron has some natural nonstick properties and can withstand very high temperatures, so it's a good pick when you're broiling. It's more expensive and a little more high maintenance than Teflon, but it's also a good long-term investment because it can last a lifetime.

File this one under "Good to know, but don't let it make you crazy." Avoid PFOAs where you can, but it's not something to freak out about.

## Microwave Popcorn

Most people don't think twice about microwaving their popcorn. It's simple and fun, right? But the coating on the bag also contains PFOA, and when you heat your popcorn and then inhale the steam from the great-smelling bag, you may be inhaling a noseful of toxins.

A safer alternative is an air popper, or popping popcorn on your stove.

# Final Thoughts

Oh, you were hoping we were going to say, "Just eat mangoes and French fries with gravy and you'll miraculously grow more eggs?" Sorry about that. There are no magical foods, but there are certainly principles about how to eat and drink to keep your fertility as strong as possible. Follow them as well as you can, while still sneaking in a little chocolate cake every now and then. Your future baby wants you to be happy.

# Chapter 8
# Preserving Your Eggs

Are you sitting down? (Of course you are—how many people read books while they're standing up?) Okay, listen up, because this is huge. It's the closest thing to a fountain of youth you can buy: It's called "egg preservation," and it literally means that some of your eggs will be removed from your ovaries and stored in a freezer. They'll stay there, not aging, while the rest of you takes your time getting ready to have a baby.

Egg preservation is neither foolproof nor a long shot; it's somewhere in between. It's also not a new thing: The first baby from a frozen egg was born in 1986. It took many years to perfect the process, though, and was not widely used in fertility clinics. The technology was not advanced enough to give women any reasonable assurance that their eggs would survive the freezing and thawing process. In the 1980s, the process usually broke open the egg membranes and damaged what was inside. Eggs have an intricate infrastructure, unlike sperm, which were always easy to freeze—plus, there are millions of sperm, so it's not as big a deal to lose some. It used to be that embryos had a much better chance of surviving a freeze cycle, but now 98.5 percent of unfertilized eggs survive this process, which is equivalent to the percentage of embryos that survive. That's a huge difference from the last decade: In 2004, just 37 percent of eggs survived.

Women whose eggs are older make embryos that are more likely to be chromosomally abnormal. That can mean no pregnancy at all, miscarriage or birth defects. So if you're not ready to have a baby in your twenties or early to mid-thirties, harvesting and freezing your eggs, if you are able to do this, is a great option. The same goes for many people who have cancer and are at risk for losing their fertility from cancer treatments.

| RISK OF DOWN SYNDROME BY MATERNAL AGE | |
| :---: | :---: |
| AGE OF MOTHER (OR HER EGGS) | RISK OF HAVING A BABY WITH DOWN SYNDROME |
| 25 | 1 in 1,300 |
| 30 | 1 in 900 |
| 35 | 1 in 350 |
| 40 | 1 in 100 |
| 42 | 1 in 60 |
| 44 | 1 in 40 |
| 47 | 1 in 20 |
| 49 | 1 in 10 |

Your age during pregnancy doesn't count for much; what really makes the difference is the age of the egg. This is something doctors realized after older women failed multiple rounds of IVF; if they used donor eggs from young, healthy women, they'd have the same pregnancy rates as young, healthy women.

Using donor eggs is still a great possibility, but many women hold tight to the hope of having their own biological children—which is where egg preservation comes into play.

# Do I Need to Do It?

When you're getting to the point where you're questioning whether or not you should do this and whether or not you need to budget for it, one of the things that may help you decide is to get antral follicle counts during your annual gynecological exams in your late twenties and thirties. That's done by transvaginal ultrasound, and it shows how many developing follicles you have, which can also provide you with an estimate of how many eggs you have remaining before your supply runs out. It doesn't tell you whether those eggs are chromosomally normal, but it does at least tell you whether you still have a significant supply or whether you're cutting it close to running out.

Having your eggs frozen is not cheap, and it's not a simple process, so most people have to weigh the pros and cons to decide if it's a viable option. What it really comes down to is this: If you lose your shot to have your own biological children, will you be crushed? Or do you think you could be happy having a child another way (such as adopting or using donor eggs)?

For Kyra's thirty-five-year-old friend Catherine, egg preservation was a huge relief. Catherine had been really stressed out about not finding the right guy in time, and Kyra convinced her to go to Jamie and freeze her eggs. At her last appointment before her egg retrieval, Catherine was nervous.

*I stared at my dangling feet and my still-fresh pedicure from the previous night with thick, opaque pink Fiji-colored toes, thinking Fiji was exactly where I wished I were. It would be warm there. I would be wiggling my toes in the moist, crumbly sand instead of in this cold, dark exam room waiting to be poked and prodded. How did I end up here? Should I have married that guy from college? We would be divorced by now, but we would have had cute, smart kids. I spent my most fertile years working for a company that never cared about me. What had I done? And how much was this exam going to hurt?*

*Dr. Grifo walked in. I liked him. He was good at putting me at ease. "Let's have a look," he said. I managed a fake smile.*

*Sure, I thought. Let's do that. If you are going to use that contraption that I think you are going to use to peer inside of me, then you might as well have a look-see at my kidneys, what I had for breakfast, my lungs and swing by my heart while you are at it.*

*After a little adjusting of me and the monitor, he said, "This is as good as it gets. You've got maybe a dozen on each side. It couldn't be better." I've always been an overachiever.*

*But he could read on my face what a lonely road this was for me. "I don't know what's wrong with men these days," he said while still examining me.*

*I couldn't hold back. Everything I thought came straight out my mouth. I can't remember if I told him how men my age won't waste a weekend on a date or that sometimes, when they find out that you have a degree higher than theirs, they find an excuse to leave in the middle of the conversation. How they will rotate you into their schedule even if they are dating someone else so they can try you on to make sure they already have the one they like and they can check you off the list once and for all. Or how they think that a booty call is a stand-in for a legitimate date. Clearly, I am surrounding myself with the wrong men. I am not sure how much of this came out, but enough of it did.*

*Dr. Grifo gave me some instructions on dosages for my injections and sent me off to get bloodwork. I put my Fiji-ed feet back on the cold linoleum floor, tiptoed off into the changing room and took a deep breath.*

*I decided to focus not on what I had just said but instead on the good news Dr. Grifo had delivered before my angry outburst. I had, potentially, twenty-four eggs. A lot of women in that room later that day would not hear this news. I needed to be grateful and respectful. No one ever said finding a good man was easy and for me that has certainly not been the case. But I will find him. And when I do, my eggs are waiting for me.*

For Catherine, the cost was worth it because it took all the pressure off. It took just one cycle, the injections were no big deal (she said they were less painful in the abdomen than in the thighs), and she didn't have any bad side effects. Now she can date without the blaring of her biological clock as the constant soundtrack.

# Picking a Clinic

When you make the decision to freeze your eggs, the first thing you need to do is pick a fertility clinic. And that's more complicated than you might think.

The problem is that not all fertility clinics have actually proven they know what they're doing with egg freezing. Some have frozen eggs, but have never actually unfrozen them, implanted them and had successful pregnancies. They're still experimenting on paying patients.

There's not just one accepted method for freezing eggs, and each lab may do it a little differently. You want to see hard data—how many times have they done egg freezing, what percentage of eggs survive the freezing and thawing processes, and what percentage of frozen eggs have resulted in live births?

Beyond percentages, ask about real numbers because percentages can be misleading. If they've thawed just one frozen egg and it resulted in a pregnancy, they can legitimately tell you they have a 100 percent success rate! But no one can sustain a number anywhere near that at this time. Neither nature nor the lab is perfect, but some labs are certainly better than others.

Jamie's lab at NYU is one of the very few with proven and published data about their success rates—they spent four years working on mice studies to practice their technique, then did a clinical study where they gave twenty-two women free egg freezing for one to four months, then thawed those eggs and performed IVF so they could test how well their technique would work on women. It was a huge success; more than half the women delivered healthy babies. It was only after that point that NYU began taking paying patients—first they wanted to prove that they knew what they were doing. Many fertility clinics are still operating without a single successful live birth following egg freezing. You need to know the numbers, and if you feel the slightest bit uncomfortable or mistrustful because they won't give you numbers, then look elsewhere.

Beyond the numbers, of course, you'll also want to find a clinic where you feel comfortable—you have to feel that you can trust your doctor, be at ease at your appointments and not have your time or money wasted. Personal recommendations are the best way to know for sure, so don't be shy about asking friends who've gone through the process how they felt about their clinic.

And while distance may have to be a consideration, don't let it be your only consideration. Kyra was living in Atlanta when she decided to work with Jamie in New York.

# The Process

The process of harvesting your eggs takes about two weeks and six to eight visits to the clinic. After bloodwork and ultrasound tests are completed to make sure everything is functioning right, you wait for day 2 of your next menstrual cycle. On that day, you start injecting yourself with medication that is meant to send your ovaries into overdrive and help you produce many mature follicles, which will develop extra eggs. Medications may include follicle-stimulating synthetic hormones, luteinizing hormones (LH) or both. Whereas normally your body would release just one egg per month, the idea here is to get it to release as many as possible so that you'll have lots of chances of future pregnancy. The average is ten eggs harvested at the end of the process. There are a few different medications that might be used, and you will inject them two or three times a day, at consistent times, into your abdomen, leg or butt.

A few days after you complete that round, you'll start injecting another medication called a GnRH agonist, which stops your body from releasing luteinizing hormone and triggering ovulation. In this case, you want to delay ovulation so all the follicles can mature.

## Jamie Says . . .

Just about all women are freaked out about the idea of the injections, but it's really not that big a deal. The idea of it is scarier than the actual experience, which is not very painful. It can leave you looking pretty black and blue, but it's just a quick prick of a needle that's done with a button, like clicking a pen. We teach patients how to do it, they hate the idea and then I rarely hear another complaint about it.

During the two weeks, you visit the clinic several times for ultrasounds (to check your ovaries) and blood tests (to check your hormone levels), and then as soon as the follicles have grown to an adequate size, you're ready for the luteinizing hormone surge.

The human chorionic gonadotropin (hCG) hormone injection finalizes the maturation of the eggs, and egg retrieval occurs just before you would ovulate from the hCG trigger. It's a precisely timed event: You'll go for the procedure thirty-five hours after you get that final shot or your ovaries will release the eggs and the retrieval will be unable to collect the eggs. You will be given intravenous anesthesia, so you need that day free. It's not the kind of thing you can plan precisely in advance; the injection happens only when your doctor says those follicles are ready for it, which doesn't happen on the same cycle day for every woman (but is around day 12 to 14 of the cycle).

On the day of "transvaginal oocyte collection," better known as egg retrieval, you can't eat or drink anything, starting at midnight before the procedure, and you'll need to have someone drive you home because you'll be groggy. During the procedure, you'll have a light anesthetic (so you'll be asleep), and then the doctor will insert a needle through your vagina and into each ovary to pull the fluid out of each developed follicle, using ultrasound to guide him. Then the fluid is given to an embryologist, who goes hunting for the eggs inside the fluid, using a microscope. The eggs are separated out and then the mature ones frozen in liquid nitrogen, where they can stay indefinitely. The whole retrieval process only takes ten to fifteen minutes.

It'll take about an hour afterwards to recover from the anesthesia, and you may have the normal side effects from it—nausea, dizziness, sleepiness and so on. You'll get an antibiotic to prevent

continued on page 152

infection. And if you have any discomfort from the procedure, you typically won't need anything stronger than simple over-the-counter pain medications and a heating pad. You may also be bloated afterwards. In some cases where the ovaries have been hyperstimulated, you may get more severe bloating and cramping for up to ten days and the ovaries may be very swollen and tender. This is called ovarian hyperstimulation syndrome (OHSS) and it's more common in women under thirty-five and those who have polycystic ovarian syndrome or very high estrogen levels during treatment. It happens only after the eggs are released. In its mild form, which can occur in about 10 percent of fertility patients, symptoms resolve on their own and don't cause any complications. In its severe form, it can cause significant weight gain (more than ten pounds within five days), shortness of breath, significant abdominal or pelvic pain, and problems urinating.

Side effects like that are rare (less than 5 percent of cases), but it's important to know that they're possible and can be severe. In my practice, hospitalization happened just a few times in 25,000 cycles.

## Kyra Says . . .

I did most of the shots in my abdomen and, for a long time, I looked like a human pincushion. You have to be diligent about doing the injections at the same time every day, but my job meant that I was often traveling on assignment in different time zones—which led to me "shooting up" in the strangest places: in the back of a car, in the airport, in public restrooms . . .

The weirdest part was when I went to get a massage and the staff all spoke Korean. My belly was all bruised and I was sure they were thinking I was being abused.

"I'm fine. I'm just doing fertility treatments!" I tried to explain, but it turns out that's not such an easy English-to-Korean translation.

## Can IVF Go Wrong?

Yes. Depending on the results of the blood tests and ultrasounds, the doctor may not let you start the process if your body conditions are not favorable. The doctor may dial down your medications if it looks like you're getting overstimulated, or she may stop the process if your body isn't responding well to the medications or if it appears you may be getting significantly overstimulated.

While there's no such thing as "too many" eggs, very high numbers of follicles and high estrogen levels indicate that you may wind up with ovarian hyperstimulation syndrome, which is dangerous if it's severe. It's also possible for you to develop internal bleeding or infection, but that rarely is serious enough to warrant hospitalization.

## What Happens After a Successful Retrieval?

When you're ready to use your eggs, you go back to the clinic for an IVF cycle. This means that some of your frozen eggs will be thawed and inspected, then combined with sperm in a petri dish. With fresh eggs, the fertility specialist can just wait and see if the sperm fertilizes the egg on its own (usually within a few hours), but the freezing process makes this impossible. Instead, they'll need to inject the sperm directly into the egg, which is called intracytoplasmic sperm injection (ICSI). Then you wait to see if it "takes"—if the egg cell gets fertilized and starts dividing. About 60–70 percent will.

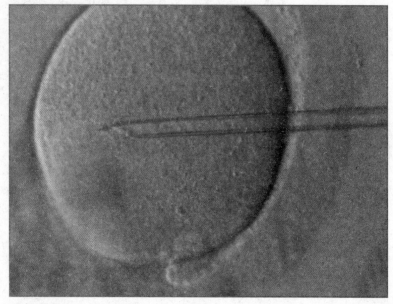

ICSI procedure

Some clinics will transfer the embryo back into the woman on day 3 of cell division, while several others (including Jamie's) wait for day 5.

While there are fewer embryos that make it to day 5 (about 50 percent of all fertilized eggs will make it), there's also a better success rate among the ones that do.

Depending on factors such as age and embryo quality, your doctor will then choose one, two or more of the most advanced embryos to implant and then refreeze any others that are viable. You'll read more about IVF in chapter 12.

---

### Do the Ovarian Stimulation Drugs "Use Up" Your Eggs?

In a word, no! Some women are concerned that making your body produce extra eggs to be harvested means that you're using up extra eggs that you'd otherwise ovulate. Not the case. Remember that each month, you lose about a thousand eggs during your menstrual cycle? These extra ovulated eggs are from those thousand. They would otherwise have just died off. You haven't used up any future candidates.

---

# Does It Work?

Until 2012, the American Society for Reproductive Medicine (ASRM) labeled egg freezing as an "experimental" treatment. It was unknown just how well the process of freezing and thawing an egg would go; it was known that freezing an embryo was effective, but just an egg?

At Jamie's clinic at NYU, which was one of the pioneers in egg freezing, their first eighty cycles using frozen eggs resulted in thirty successful pregnancies and four miscarriages. That's just about the same success rate as regular IVF using fresh eggs. This was so shocking to people in the field that he had trouble getting a peer-reviewed journal to publish his findings—doctors just wouldn't believe that you could get the same results from thawed eggs as from fresh eggs. He was even accused of fabricating his results, even though the results were mostly crawling around in diapers by then.

Unsurprisingly, success rates are better when the woman freezing her eggs is younger—although there are always exceptions. The rates of multiples (twins, triplets, etc.) is also similar with frozen eggs and typical IVF—21 percent and 25 percent, respectively, as of 2013. These numbers will likely go down as genetic testing becomes more and more common and doctors are able to implant just one genetically sound embryo (called a "euploid" embryo) at a time.

In cases that don't involve medical necessity, Jamie suggests that the right time to freeze your eggs is in your early thirties. There's no need to do it before then because you really don't know where your life is headed—at twenty-one, you still have many years before you have to start worrying that you haven't found the right guy or haven't gotten financially stable. By your early thirties, you'll have a better idea of your life trajectory and whether or not you're headed for the fertility danger zone.

While egg freezing is a wonderful new way to add years to your fertility, it's not foolproof, so go into it keeping those success rates in mind—not all eggs are healthy enough to freeze and not all viable eggs result in a pregnancy. Because it's still a recent technology, we also don't know for sure if eggs deteriorate over time in storage. We don't think they do. Just as with airplane flights, the danger is primarily in take-off and landing. That's the case with eggs, too—the danger is in the freezing and thawing, but once they're frozen, they're stable. There are cases where eggs that have been frozen for ten years have resulted in successful pregnancies, and Jamie has cases in his clinic where embryos have resulted in pregnancies after fifteen years.

# The Cost

On average across the country, it costs about $8,000 for one round of egg retrieval, plus the cost of medications, which can run you another $3,000 to $5,000. The first year of storage is usually included in the cost; after that, you'll pay several hundred dollars a year to keep your eggs frozen. Prices vary, depending on where you live.

Then, when you're ready to use your eggs, there will be a separate fee to go through IVF, and that can cost about $5,000, including medications. Unless you're freezing your eggs to preserve your fertility before cancer treatments, insurance typically will not cover any of this cost.

Ideally, you will do more than one round. You want to get as many eggs in that freezer as possible, so it depends on how your body produces—you might get a dozen or more eggs in one round, or it might be just six or seven. Most likely, not all of them will survive the freezing and thawing process, and not all will be chromosomally normal. So it can be worrisome to realize that you have just one or two viable eggs at the end of your round.

For most women, however, the cost is a major factor. It may be that if you can afford it at all, one round is all you can do. And that's okay; any insurance toward your future fertility is better than none. The technology is advancing so quickly in this area, and all you really need is one great egg to take advantage of it!

# Chapter 9
# BMI and Fertility

We know that you don't need any extra reasons to feel bad about your body if you're not the "perfect" weight, but here's the simple truth: Being too underweight or overweight can make you infertile and can cause problems during pregnancy.

## Calculating Your BMI

A healthy body mass index (BMI) is 18.5 to 24.9. You can ask your doctor at your next checkup, or you can weigh yourself and do some simple math:

**The formula is: weight (lb) / [height (in)]$^2$ x 703**

Wait! Don't worry! It's simpler than it looks. First, figure out your height in inches. Let's say you're 67 inches tall. Square that—so, 67 times 67. You get 4,489. Now figure out your weight—let's say 140 pounds—and divide your weight by that height-squared number (140 divided by 4,489 is 0.03118734 . . . ). Well, we don't need to go that far into the decimals! We can stick to just

0.031. Now multiply that number by 703, and you get 21.793. Good going! Imaginary you is in the right range.

If the math still hurts your brain, then just go online and search for a BMI calculator. There are plenty of them. Just don't cheat. We all have those scales that may be calibrated just a bit in our favor, by sheer accident, of course.

# Underweight

Whether you're underweight or overweight, your BMI can help to predict how fertile you'll be. Your BMI is a number that takes into account your height and weight, to determine whether you're in an optimal range, too low or too high. It's estimated that up to 12 percent of infertility patients have low weight or overexercise as a contributing factor.

You may have a very healthy-looking physique, but if you're a serious athlete, then you most likely have very little fat on your body—too little fat for fertility purposes. Any BMI under 18.5, which is the low end of what's considered normal, is dangerously low for fertility.

Beyond BMI, you can also check your body fat percentage, which should be between 12 percent and 30 percent. You can use calipers to measure this. (You squeeze a pinch of your skin and fat and then use a metal device, called "skin fold calipers," to determine how much body fat you have. You can buy the device and see videos online to show you how to use it, or have measurements done at a gym or a doctor's office.) It's possible to have an acceptable BMI, but still have body fat that's too low for fertility.

If you're not in the proper body fat range, you typically stop ovulating. Your body figures that it can't support a pregnancy, so why try? The good news is that most athletes can restore their fertility within just a few months by cutting down on their training and easing up on their diets. This is not always true, however, and cycles can be affected for longer spans.

If you're doing vigorous exercise for more than an hour a day, you're overdoing it for fertility purposes. Your body starts shutting down the hormones that help your ovaries function. So when you're getting ready to start trying to conceive, ease up.

Jamie has also had patients who were underweight for different reasons.

"I can't help but notice that you look very thin," he said to one of them. "Do you have any problems with your eating?"

"Yes," she said. "I'm in treatment for bulimia."

She was there to try IVF, but he knew that it wouldn't work until she had her underlying problem resolved. He encouraged her to finish her treatment first and get her eating disorder under control so that her body would start ovulating on its own again and be able to sustain a pregnancy.

Pregnancy can also exacerbate existing eating disorders simply because you will gain weight during pregnancy. For some people with eating disorders, this is a problem and they'll starve themselves, binge and purge, take diet pills, or overexercise to deal with it. It's probably obvious to state that this is no good for the baby or the mom and puts both their lives in danger. For those reasons and many others, it's important to get treated for eating disorders before you try to get pregnant. There is effective help out there. You may want to start your search at www.nationaleatingdisorders.org, a national nonprofit group to support people with eating disorders.

Even if you don't have an eating disorder, but you're just naturally skinny, it will likely still affect your ovarian function if you fall below normal BMI and body fat thresholds.

# Overweight

More common than being underweight, however, is being overweight. We all know that we're in the midst of an obesity epidemic in America, and this may have a lot to do with the fact that our fertility rates are also declining. It is estimated that being overweight is a factor in about 25 percent of infertility cases, but the good news is that even a small loss of weight can have a big impact on your fertility.

You're considered overweight if your BMI falls between 25 and 29.9, and obese if your BMI is 30 or above. In the United States now, more than one in three adults is obese. It's no fun to hear this label applied to yourself, particularly if you thought you just had a few pounds to lose, but it's an important wake-up call for your health and your future.

It's so important to get yourself in shape before trying to have a baby, whether that's in the bedroom or at a fertility clinic. You're much more likely to have a positive outcome either way if you can get your BMI into a healthy range.

There's more than one way that being overweight can harm your fertility. It can lead to ovulatory problems and irregular menstrual cycles, but not necessarily in the ways you might expect. When eggs were compared between women who were obese, overweight and healthy weight, there were no significant differences in the quality of the eggs—they had about the same levels of genetic abnormalities. The problem didn't seem to be with the eggs, but with the environment the eggs had to live in. Excess weight is also highly associated with PCOS—more than 60 percent of women with PCOS are overweight, which can be a chicken-or-egg question because PCOS can make people gain weight. Losing weight can lessen the severity of the condition.

In a large-scale study of close to 10,000 women undergoing IVF treatments using donor eggs, in which all the donor women were of normal weight, researchers analyzed whether the BMI of the egg recipients mattered to the outcome. It turned out to be very linear; as BMI went up, outcomes got worse. Overweight and obese women had more trouble with implantation and holding onto a pregnancy.[1]

"Based on our results, the chance of having a baby by egg donation is reduced by around one-third for obese women," said Dr. Jose Bellver of the Valencia Infertility Institute in Spain. "We found that obese recipients of eggs from normal-weight donors had a 23 percent lower implantation rate than normal-weight recipients, a 19 percent lower clinical pregnancy rate and a 27 percent lower live-birth rate."

Because there have been several studies showing worse pregnancy outcomes for obese women, whether they're going through unassisted pregnancy or fertility treatments, clinics in some other countries won't even accept women with BMIs that are considered too high. The women are advised to lose weight before starting treatments.

## Gastric Bypass Surgery

If you're considering weight-loss surgery and wondering what it would mean for you in terms of childbearing, there are two important facts to keep in mind. Yes, it normally does help with fertility. Not only do most women who get the surgery get a big bump in their ability to ovulate normally, but it also often resolves PCOS. And as far as safety afterwards, it's safe to get pregnant after surgery as long as you wait about eighteen months. Those first eighteen months are when the major weight loss happens and you'd be at risk of malnourishing a developing fetus while you're in this state. After weight-loss surgery, provided you attain a healthy weight, you have the same risk of gestational diabetes and hypertension as a person who's never been obese.

# Insulin Resistance

One of the major problems with being overweight is that your body no longer processes insulin correctly. Here's what it's supposed to do:

After you eat, some of your food is converted in the small intestine into the simple sugar glucose, which is delivered all over your body to provide energy to your organs. You need that energy to do everything you do all day long—walk, talk, think, digest, breathe, and so on. In order for your organs to use that glucose, though, they need a helper: insulin. The pancreas produces the hormone insulin and sends it out along with the glucose. What the insulin does is act like a key: The cells are "locked" until insulin shows up, unlocks the cells and lets them know that it's time to accept some glucose.

The pancreas sends out just the right amount of insulin to unlock the right number of cells, depending on how much glucose there is.

However, this can go wrong in three main ways: type 1 diabetes, type 2 diabetes and insulin resistance.

In type 1 diabetes, the body attacks cells in the pancreas, which then loses the ability to produce insulin at all. In type 2 diabetes (which is associated with being overweight), the pancreas still produces insulin, but not enough. Typically, a person will need to lose weight, make dietary and lifestyle changes, and/or take supplemental insulin to deal with this problem.

Insulin resistance is related to diabetes, but it's not the same thing. A person with type 2 diabetes may develop insulin resistance, but a person doesn't need to be diabetic in order to have this condition. It does happen most often to people who are overweight or obese, though. With this problem, insulin is still produced, but the body no longer processes it correctly—it doesn't "unlock" the cells the way it should. It works ineffectively, with just some of the insulin still able to unlock the cells and the rest of the insulin just floating around helplessly with the glucose.

As a result, the pancreas tries to compensate by producing more and more insulin. It overdoes the insulin like crazy in the hopes that some of it will work—but it can't keep up. That means that there's lots of extra glucose that's just staying in the bloodstream instead of reaching the organs all over the body, where it's supposed to go. The organs aren't getting their energy, and the blood is getting oversugared. This is what it means when you hear the term "high blood sugar," or hyperglycemia. It means that there's too much glucose floating around and not enough insulin (or not effectively working insulin) carrying it where it needs to go. Generally, if you're hyperglycemic, you're also insulin-resistant.

The most common symptoms of hyperglycemia are frequent or excessive thirst, needing to urinate a lot, blurred vision, feeling weak or tired, and having dry skin. Occasional mild hyperglycemia is usually not a big deal—it may not even have symptoms. But long term, it can lead to major health consequences, ranging from blindness to kidney problems.

Insulin resistance also sets you up for metabolic syndrome, which is associated with a higher risk of heart disease and diabetes.

## What Does Insulin Resistance Have to Do with Fertility?

High insulin levels—a condition that occurs if your pancreas is over-compensating and sending out more insulin—cause your ovaries and adrenal glands to make more male hormones. You really don't want extra testosterone when you're trying to make a baby. It may surprise you to find out that you have any testosterone at all, but women's bodies make about 10 percent as much testosterone as men's do. You need testosterone to boost your sex drive and for healthy muscles and bones. Conversely, men also need to produce some estrogen. But when it comes to babymaking, extra male hormones interfere with your ability to ovulate properly. (And on the flip side of that coin, men who are obese produce less testosterone and frequently have erectile dysfunction. Low testosterone can often be treated with Clomid or other medications.)

Women who are insulin-resistant are statistically much more likely to have recurrent miscarriages and to have fertility treatments fail.

## So What Can I Do About It?

Well, you probably already have an idea of what needs to happen here if you suspect you are overweight, and particularly if you've developed insulin resistance. In short, you need to change your diet and exercise habits. Forget crash diets, fad diets, diet pills and the like—for your body to have a chance to recover and begin using hormones appropriately again, you need to make substantial lifestyle changes.

The nutrition chapter ("Eat, Drink and Be Fertile") gives you a strong starting point about the type of diet you should adopt. As far as exercise goes, half an hour at least three times a week is a good start. If you're not up to running around for half an hour at once just yet, that's okay—we now know you can break it up into three ten-minute increments and derive the same benefit. So bike to work instead of driving, take the stairs instead of the elevator, take on a side business as a dog walker, join a yoga class, pick up a Zumba DVD, learn to belly dance, jog with a friend . . . whatever you want to try, whatever feels fun to you, do it. Heck, you can take pole dancing classes if you're feeling sassy.

The more important question is this: "How will I keep myself on track?" It's very easy to promise to make a change, and fairly easy to get started—but without the motivation to keep yourself going, it can be very difficult to see lasting results.

Here are a few tips for making these important changes in your life:

- **BE ACCOUNTABLE.** It can help a great deal to join in some kind of fitness community—like a weight-loss challenge, where you have to check in with one another. On a day when you might otherwise have said, "Screw it, I'll have the cake," knowing that you have to weigh in or report to somebody the next day can keep you on your better behavior. Another way to keep yourself honest is to have a buddy walk or jog with you. Pick someone who won't bail easily—preferably someone who's already into fitness. Make a point of meeting each other every day or two at a predetermined time—after breakfast or after work/school.

- **KEEP A FOOD JOURNAL.** You might be shocked when you are forced to write down and look at everything you consume in a day. All the times you grab a "little snack" add up! A helpful tool you can use is www.fitday.com. There, not only can you keep a food journal, but you can easily see the nutrition information about each food item, get an idea of what percentage of protein, carbs, fats and alcohol you're consuming in a day, what your daily calorie count is, how many calories you're burning by exercise and what you need to do each day to make sure you're burning more calories than you're consuming. It can be a huge eye-opener.

"I knew that a diet high in carbs was no good, and I suspected that might have been my problem, but until I actually saw it on a chart, I had no idea that about 80 percent of my daily diet was carbs!" said Kayla. "I really just didn't know what qualified as carbs . . . I thought only bread and pasta and potatoes did. I wasn't big into junk food, so I thought I was eating pretty healthy. No wonder I couldn't take the weight off."

After charting for a couple of weeks, she got into a routine of eating lots more salads and lean meat and dropped twelve pounds within two months, improving her odds of fertility.

- **GET "BAD FOODS" OUT OF THE HOUSE.** It's so much easier not to give in to temptation if the temptation isn't sitting right there in your cabinet. If you live with someone, try to get that person onboard, too. If that isn't feasible, ask the other person to keep tempting snacks hidden from you. A locked safe would be fine!

- **MAKE A VISION BOARD OR SOME OTHER VISUAL REMINDER.** A vision board is a piece of tag or poster board where you make a visual representation of the things you want in your life. In this case, you might want to write down your goal weight or just a picture of a woman exercising or looking fit, along with a picture of a baby or some other representation of your hope for a future pregnancy. Remind yourself visually of why you're doing this each day. It's not just about how you look in skinny jeans; there's a larger purpose.

- **DON'T BE TOO STRICT.** Never allowing yourself a piece of birthday cake or an occasional cheat is a recipe for failure for most people. You're not training for the Olympics; you're trying to get to a healthy weight so that your body will work at its peak. Work hard, eat right and do your best—but allow yourself to be human, too, so that you don't hate the process so much that you give it up because it's too hard.

- **CELEBRATE YOUR VICTORIES.** Depending on how far you have to go, you might want to treat yourself at certain intervals—maybe every ten pounds. Obviously, don't treat yourself with food! You don't want to associate junk food with rewards. But maybe treat yourself to a manicure, a massage, a new pair of jeans (you'll need them!) or a movie.

Once you're pregnant, don't let that become an excuse to give up your healthier habits. Remember that the baby is essentially eating whatever you're eating, so whole fruits and veggies are better than deep-fried Oreos! It'll also put you on track for a healthy pregnancy, reduce your risk of gestational diabetes and preeclampsia (a very serious condition for both you and your baby that can force you to deliver early), and reduce the risk of your child having autism (a recent study of a thousand children in California showed that moms who were obese during pregnancy had a 67 percent higher risk of having a child with autism).[2]

Of course, it'll also make it a lot easier for you to get rid of the pregnancy weight afterwards if you don't gain too much. Some of it is beyond your control (like our friend Beth, who just had a ton of amniotic fluid and gained thirty-seven pounds despite eating healthfully—she also lost all thirty-seven pounds easily afterwards because it was all baby and fluid!).

You don't need to strive for perfection, but do your best to usher your body into those healthy BMI numbers. You can totally do it. Rock on.

# Chapter 10
# Rumors, Myths and Truths about Fertility

When it comes to fertility, there's no shortage of old wives' tales, rumors and just plain bad advice rooted in misinformation. We'll address some of the most persistent and quirkiest myths and give you the real scoop.

## Standing in front of a microwave will make you infertile.

### MYTH.

There's a constant fear that standing near microwaves causes infertility. The only real reason you'd have to worry is if the microwave door hinges, latch or seal was damaged and allowed radiation to leak out. In that case, get a new one. Microwaves also have to pass safety inspections that allow for very little radiation to leak—levels far below what have ever been shown to hurt people. And you'd have to basically be standing an inch or two away from the microwave to even get that minute exposure.

The FDA says not to bother with devices meant to test your microwave for leaks: Most of them have been shown to be inaccurate. As long as your microwave is intact, don't worry about it.

## TV/computers make you sterile.

### MYTH...MOSTLY.

There was a study done in 2013 at Harvard showing that men who watched a lot of television (more than twenty hours per week) had 44 percent less sperm than men who didn't watch TV.[1] But does that mean that the television is giving off some mysterious sperm-poisoning ray? No, it most likely means that those TV-watchers are more sedentary, more overweight and less likely to exercise, all of which we know to be factors in both male and female fertility. The study showed a direct correlation between lack of physical activity and lowered sperm counts and concentrations (and vice versa—men in the highest category of physical activity had the highest sperm concentration).

## Bacon harms fertility.

### MAYBE.

Presenters at the American Society for Reproductive Medicine annual meeting in 2013 showed a study that linked processed meat consumption (at least half a serving a day) with poorer sperm parameters—lowered sperm concentrations and more abnormally shaped sperm. There's a lot to consider before leaping on that train of thought, however. First, it was a small study of 156 men undergoing IVF. The researchers also found that men who ate fish regularly had better sperm. But before we say that bacon causes infertility, we have to consider the many other factors that go into that possibility: Aside from bacon, what's the diet like for the rest of these men? Are they eating fresh fruits and vegetables? Are they overweight and inactive?

We know by now that processed meats (such as bacon, sausage and hamburger) are bad for you, and that they are linked with all kinds of problems, such as heart disease and colon cancer. But as far as whether or not they're linked with infertility for men or women, the research is inconclusive at this point. We advocate a commonsense approach. Look, if you love bacon and sausage, you don't have to cut them out of your life entirely. But think of them as rare treats, not staple foods.

# If you want to have a baby, just relax and go on vacation.

## MOSTLY A MYTH.

Although there are plenty of anecdotal stories of people getting pregnant on vacation, there's very little evidence that stress has anything to do with infertility. It can be very frustrating for people who are going through infertility to hear others say, "Oh, it's because you're so stressed out about it! Just relax!" Nonsense. Eggs don't suddenly get more genetically normal because you're at the beach.

That said, we don't want to knock the idea of stress reduction. There have been some small studies showing that stress-reduction exercises have improved the odds for people going through IVF. To be sure, it's a great goal to reduce stress; even if we don't know that it will affect your fertility directly, it does affect your health and happiness—but the problem is that it can be a vicious cycle when you feel pressured to reduce your stress! If adding a meditation class to your schedule is just going to make you feel as if that's one more thing you have to squeeze in, then don't do it. It'll be counterproductive. Find little ways to relax in the manner that best suits you—take walks, go swimming, listen to guided meditations, take a nap in the sun, whatever you find calming.

## Certain sex positions will help you conceive.

### MYTH.

Sorry, nope. Sex is sex as far as conception is concerned. As long as you're in the right orifice, you're solid.

## Winter is the most popular time to conceive.

### FACT.

More babies are born in fall than in any other season, which means that most conceptions happen in winter and early spring. People assume that's because we stay indoors more in the cold months and have less to do, so we tend to have more sex then. That's probably part of the story, but a new study of more than six thousand semen samples over the course of three years may provide the other part of the story: Sperm swim faster and are shaped better in the winter, and their concentrations are higher, too.[2]

## You're more likely to get pregnant after you adopt.

### MYTH.

Sure, there are cases when this has happened, but you're no more likely to get pregnant after you adopt than before you adopt. This is a variation on the myth that stress is what's causing women not to get pregnant, the idea being that once you've adopted, you're no longer stressed out about wanting a child.

## You have a better chance of getting pregnant if you put your legs up after sex.

### MYTH.

By the time you're done having sex, the sperm are already where they need to be. Putting your legs up or putting a pillow under your butt doesn't help. But if it makes you feel that you're being proactive, then go right ahead!

## You can use a turkey baster to inseminate yourself.

### FACT.

Well, you can, but it's simpler to use an oral medicine syringe (or any needleless syringe). Many women who use donor sperm choose to do this at home rather than going through artificial insemination at a clinic. The man collects his semen in a clean cup, you draw it into the syringe and then insert it as close to the cervix as possible. At a clinic, they'd more likely do IUI (intrauterine insemination), which gets the sperm right into your uterus as opposed to your vagina, so the odds of success are greater.

## You should have sex every day if you want to get pregnant.

### MYTH.

Having sex every day (or multiple times a day) doesn't actually boost your chances. Every other day up to the time of ovulation is fine. That gives the sperm time to build up again. When you have sex more often than that, it dilutes the concentration of sperm in the seminal fluid. Your odds are best if you have sex within two days before ovulation. It's better to have the sperm already there waiting when the egg makes its glorious debut, rather than waiting until ovulation has occurred. Sperm can live for several days, so it's okay to leave them hanging there for a bit while your egg is primping for its date.

## Take baby aspirin to help you conceive.

### UNCLEAR.

Because aspirin has anti-inflammatory and anticoagulant effects, researchers have surmised that it could help blood flow to the uterus when you're trying to conceive. Multiple studies have been conducted to find out if a low dose of aspirin helps in any manner—if it helps women conceive, hold onto a pregnancy, reduce the risk of complications and so on, and the results have been largely contradictory, skewing toward the idea that the aspirin has little to no effect.

However, in one large, multiyear study, it was shown that among women who'd had a miscarriage in the last year, taking daily low-dose aspirin was associated with faster positive pregnancy tests and clinically confirmed pregnancies. Researchers said they weren't sure if the aspirin was helping women get pregnant faster or helping to prevent very early miscarriages. But the effect was seen only in that subset of women, not in women who'd had more than one miscarriage.

Since there are few side effects of baby aspirin, and because it can help with various other issues, such as blood clots, many fertility doctors tell their patients to take it during parts of treatment and early pregnancy.

## You get hornier when you're ovulating.

### FACT.

Not only are you programmed to want more sex when you're ovulating but you're also more likely to be attracted to more stereotypically "manly men" during that time of your cycle—taller guys with strong jawlines, deeper voices, bigger physiques and those who have higher levels of testosterone. You're also more likely to dress in a sexier way and buy sexy clothes during your most fertile times of the month. It's just evolution's way of making sure you get out there and carry on our species. No pressure or anything.

## You're more likely to get pregnant if you have an orgasm.

### FACT.

The muscle contractions you get when you orgasm help to pull the sperm into the cervix and closer to the egg. Biologists Robin Baker and Mark Bellis tested this idea by asking volunteers to record the timing of their orgasms and then checking the fluids that came out of the vagina after sex.[3] What they found was that the woman retained much more sperm if she had an orgasm between one minute before the man ejaculated and forty-five minutes afterwards. It didn't help if her orgasm came more than a minute before his.

Of course, you don't have to orgasm to get pregnant. It just helps a little. So if you're trying to get pregnant and the big O doesn't happen, you can have you partner stimulate or masturbate you after he finishes if you want to increase your chances.

## A woman can't get pregnant again if she's breast-feeding.

### MYTH.

Typically, women who are breast-feeding don't get their periods back as soon as women who aren't. But that's not always the case—we know an unlucky woman who got her period back nine days after giving birth, even though she was breast-feeding! Prolactin, the hormone associated with making milk, generally suppresses the hormones you need to ovulate, so it's true that most women don't ovulate for the first several months after they start breast-feeding. Even so, if you want to protect yourself from getting pregnant again too quickly, use birth control while breast-feeding.

## Donating your eggs uses up your supply.

## MYTH.

Donating eggs uses the same egg-retrieval process as we described earlier, which requires you to go through a strict course of medications and injections. But don't let your future fertility be a concern; it doesn't use up your egg supply. It just uses up some of the eggs that your body was going to lose that cycle anyway. Instead of maturing one egg and having your body throw away 999 others that month, maybe you'll mature twelve eggs and throw away 988 instead.

# Chapter 11
# When You're Ready to Start Trying

Considering how many accidental pregnancies there are, you'd think that getting pregnant was a pretty simple thing to do. Your mom probably gave you that talk quite some time ago. "When two people fall in love..."

And for some people, it is simple. But let's say that you are ready for a baby now and you want the best chances for making that happen. There are some things you should know.

## The Rhythm Method

If you've heard about the "rhythm method" as a method of contraception, what you've probably heard is that it doesn't work and you shouldn't rely on it. Well, it's true that you shouldn't rely on it because every woman's cycle is different and it's not as simple as saying, "You're fertile only on days 10–14 of your cycle." For starters, some women have textbook-perfect twenty-eight-day cycles and others have cycles that are much longer or shorter. And even the "perfect" cases ovulate on different days within their cycle, so there's no formula that can tell you exactly when you can and can't conceive.

But...

That doesn't mean it's all just a willy-nilly guessing game, either. To start, there are some days you can conceive and some days you can't. It's not technically impossible to conceive while you have your period, for instance, but it's super-unlikely. That's because the only way you can get pregnant is if there is sperm in the fallopian tube at the same time that your egg is hanging out there—which lasts for just about twenty-four hours after the egg is released from the ovary. Then the window is over. Sperm can live in the woman's reproductive tract for about three days (possibly even up to six days), so you don't have to have intercourse on that one "perfect" day when you ovulate, but it has to be reasonably close. There are about four days out of each month, in total, when you have a good chance of getting pregnant.

It's theoretically possible that you can get pregnant while you're still menstruating, but only if you have a very short cycle. Let's say you have a twenty-four-day cycle and you ovulate on day 10 of your cycle. You have a seven-day period (unlucky you), and you have sex on the last day of your period. Some of the sperm survives for three days, so it's still there during that window when you ovulate, soon after your period ends, and presto, you have an embryo.

On average, though, women ovulate about fourteen days before their next period starts, which is too far after the last period ends for period-sex to wind up getting us pregnant. So, depending on your "schedule," you might want to just try having sex a bunch around that time—midway through your cycle—and see how it turns out. Just figure out how long your cycle is by writing down when your period starts for two months in a row, and then count fourteen days backwards from when your next period is scheduled to start. But if you want the odds stacked more in your favor, there are ways for you to determine when you're most fertile.

# Basal Thermometer

One of the best tools for this is a basal thermometer—not a regular thermometer—which you can buy online for under $20. A basal thermometer is specifically used for determining when you're most fertile, and is accurate to one-tenth of a degree. That's important because the differences in temperature that you're going to be looking for are minute—less than one degree.

Your basal body temperature (BBT) is the lowest temperature you'll have all day. It generally happens first thing in the morning before you get out of bed. Your BBT should be consistent throughout the month (about 97.0–97.5°F) except the day or two after you ovulate, when it will go up just a small amount—one- or two-tenths of a degree, most likely. So it won't help you to learn your BBT that first month, because by the time the uptick happens, it's already likely too late to get pregnant that cycle—but it helps you plan future cycles.

Starting on day 1 of your menstrual cycle (the first day of your period), take your temperature while you're still lying in bed every morning at the same time. That's pretty easy to do if you have a regular schedule for work or school that requires you to get up at the same time every day. But if not, set an alarm for the same time every morning, take your temperature, write it down and then go back to sleep.

If your uptick in temperature happened on day 15 of your cycle, then you know you ovulated on day 13 or 14. If it happened on day 13, then you ovulated on day 11 or 12, and so on.

You should quickly see a pattern. Most women ovulate on approximately the same cycle day every month if their periods are regular. So, let's say you find out you normally ovulate on cycle day 11. That means your fertility window is really cycle days 8, 9, 10 and 11, so that's when you should have all the sex.

# Cervical Mucus

Here's one of those things you probably never thought about before you thought about your fertility. The consistency of your cervical mucus can tell you when you're most fertile, and it can also help or hinder your odds of conception.

Unlike your BBT, which can tell you this only after you've ovulated, the consistency of your cervical mucus can tell you when you're about to ovulate. It varies throughout the month, but when you're most fertile, it'll be wet and stretchy, with the consistency of a raw egg white. There's even an acronym for it: EWCM (egg white cervical mucus). After you've ovulated, it'll turn sticky or dry and there will be much less of it.

So how do you check your cervical mucus? Well, get in touch with yourself, girl! With your (clean, duh) fingers, you can just go ahead and reach right in there and check. Rub a little of it between your thumb and middle finger or index finger and see how it stretches. If it breaks right away, you're probably not ovulating, but if it's thin and you can stretch it a couple of inches, you're probably at your most fertile.

This type of cervical mucus helps sperm survive and make it through the reproductive tract, so it's good to have a lot of it. If it's too scant or acidic, that hurts sperm on their journey.

Some women never have EWCM, or have very little of it just for one day a month. That can hurt your chances of getting those spermies where they need to be. Here are some things that can mess up your cervical mucus:

- Antihistamines
- Smoking
- Some antidepressants (ask your doctor)
- Dehydration
- High doses of vitamin C (several grams daily)
- Infections

- Aging
- Douching (didn't we already tell you to quit douching?)
- Vaginal lubricant
- Antiseizure medications
- Clomid (even though Clomid is a fertility drug to promote ovulation, it can also decrease the quality of your cervical mucus)

The only lubricant made for those who are trying to conceive (TTC) is Preseed, which you can buy online or at drugstores. It's meant to mimic fertile cervical fluids and it won't harm sperm. Although it stops short of claiming to actually aid fertility, lots of women swear by it—check the Amazon reviews and you'll see how many people believe it was the key to their getting pregnant. It comes in a box with applicators if you want to insert it internally, or you can just use it externally, too.

To improve your cervical mucus, here are some things you can try:

- **WATER:** Make sure you're staying hydrated. By the same token, cut back on caffeine and soda, both of which can dehydrate you. Back off the Diet Coke, lady.

- **EXPECTORANTS:** Cough medicines that have guaifenesin as the only active ingredient can help. Guaifenesin helps to thin and increase mucus production when you have a cough, but guess where it also works? In your hoo-ha! Just make absolutely sure that there are no other active ingredients. You don't want to take anything with antihistamines, decongestants or cough suppressants when you're trying to conceive, as those can hurt your chances.

- **EVENING PRIMROSE OIL:** There are no scientific studies about this yet, but again, many women enthusiastically report that a daily capsule of evening primrose oil (which is made from the seeds of a wildflower) improves their EWCM.

It's not recommended during pregnancy, however (it might cause uterine contractions), so make sure to stop taking it after you ovulate each cycle.

- **Baby carrots:** Another remedy that gets tossed around quite a bit in TTC circles is baby carrots. Baby carrots are immature carrots, whereas baby-cut carrots are just bigger, uglier carrots that have been cut into pretty little pieces and sometimes washed in chlorine. No scientific studies back up carrots as a fertility aid but, at worst, you've eaten a bunch of healthy vegetables and it didn't get you pregnant. So you've been tricked into getting extra vitamins. Curses!

# Ovulation Test Kits

Ovulation predictor kits are just like pregnancy tests, except that you pee on a stick to find out whether or not you're ovulating. You have to pee on a stick every day around the time you're most likely to ovulate until you get a positive result, which can get costly, but it's also a pretty simple way of finding out when it's that magical time.

The test accomplishes this by measuring your luteinizing hormone (LH): When it surges, you're typically about thirty-six hours away from ovulating. Some tests also measure your estrogen level.

You can get these kits at drugstores, online or even in grocery stores.

# To Chart or Not to Chart

There are at least two types of women who are TTC: those who like to chart and those who don't. For some, it gives us a sense of control and something productive we can do to increase our fertility odds. For others, it makes us focus even more every day on the singular quest to make a baby, which can get too obsessive. It can also make sex too "scheduled." You've seen the movie scenes where the woman is taking her temperature and then calls the guy at work and makes him come home in the middle of a meeting for some babymaking nookie. (First of all, that's just ineffective. If your temperature has risen, it's too late. Secondly, your real window of opportunity is not that narrow that you'd ever need to drop what you're doing right now and get nekkid.)

You just need to figure out which type you are. If charting makes you feel good, do it. If it makes you feel bad, cut it out.

# Correcting the Problems

There are other things you should try before resorting to fertility treatments, assuming you're not too crunched for time.

## Quit Your Bad Habits

Quit smoking, don't drink to excess, don't do drugs, get your BMI into the proper range and do what you can to keep your body healthy. It's common sense, but a body that's in healthy condition has better odds of conceiving.

## Get Some Sleep

Getting eight hours of sleep (approximately) is always good advice, but when you're TTC, it's particularly good advice. When you don't get enough sleep, your body doesn't make enough leptin, which is an essential hormone for ovulation (and helps regulate your appetite, too). In fact, when athletes with ultra-low body fat who weren't menstruating were given leptin supplements, they got their periods back.

So getting enough sleep is important, but so is getting sleep during the right hours. Working a night shift or swing shifts is not good for your fertility. It throws off your circadian rhythms and can make your menstrual cycles irregular. It's like living in a constant state of jet lag and your body loses its natural cues about when to eat, sleep and even ovulate.

## De-Stress

Do what you can to alleviate stress in your life. Stress is sometimes unfairly . . . er, stressed when fertility comes up. "You're trying too hard. Forget all these charts and calendars. Just take a vacation and it'll happen!" people will say ever so helpfully. Yet so rarely do these people offer to pay for your vacations or stand in for you at work. Which is why these people should be hit in the face with pies.

Seriously, it helps no one when people order us to relax. You know what it makes us feel?

"I MUST RELAX IMMEDIATELY. WHY AM I NOT RELAXING? I'M FAILING AT RELAXING. THIS IS WHY I CAN'T GET PREGNANT, BECAUSE I SUCK AT BEING CALM. RELAX NOW, DAMMIT! FOR THE LOVE OF ALL THAT IS HOLY, FIND INNER PEACE NOW!"

The truth is that stressed-out people get pregnant plenty, and you don't have to get into some kind of Zen state to have sperm meet egg. But it's also true that stress doesn't help, and there have been multiple studies showing that stress can be a factor in fertility.

A study of 818 couples at fertility clinics in Denmark showed that women who reported more marital stress related to infertility took an average of three fertility treatment cycles to conceive, whereas those who reported less marital stress took an average of two cycles to conceive.[1]

Similarly, researchers at the University of San Diego found that women who reported higher levels of stress had a tougher time with egg retrieval: There were fewer eggs retrieved and fewer eggs fertilized per cycle among those who reported being the most stressed out.[2]

But don't let those studies stress you out! The good news is that techniques to alleviate stress do seem to work. A recent study of 143 women at a fertility clinic in Boston divided the women into two groups: One group went to a ten-session mind-body program meant to alleviate stress and the other group didn't. In the second cycle, 52 percent of the mind-body group got pregnant, compared to 20 percent of the control group.

One of the potential ways to alleviate stress is acupuncture, which has pretty solid evidence showing it promotes fertility. There are at least three studies showing that acupuncture improves pregnancy rates among IVF patients, and when several studies were pooled together, researchers found that, overall, adding acupuncture boosted pregnancy rates in an IVF cycle from about 35 percent to about 45 percent.

Acupuncture is a strange sort of thing—a practitioner inserts several tiny needles under the skin in strategic places and then has you just lie there for a while. Some people believe in it, others think it's wacko nonsense, but it's been shown to have positive results in everything from cancer treatment to addiction management. It might just be relaxing (you're forced to lie still for a while and listen to soothing music), or it might be that it increases blood flow to the uterus and opens the cervix. No one can definitely explain why acupuncture may improve the odds of conception, only that it does seem to help some people.

## Kyra Says . . .

I had mixed experiences with acupuncture. I'd done it a few times before, so when I was starting fertility treatments, I was open to trying it again. I knew it didn't hurt and could be relaxing, at least. Unfortunately, this time was totally different from my prior experiences.

It was a cold, sterile room that felt like a doctor's office. The acupuncturist was matter-of-fact and didn't seem to have a lot of confidence. She started sticking me, then covered me in a bizarre tin-foil blanket and left the room. I freaked the heck out. I had a panic attack and began yanking the needles out and left.

Ambience is important. Check out the facility and the feel of the place. You want to be treated in a soothing, spiritual environment—it's not supposed to make you feel more tense than when you came in!

## Stay Optimistic

This one goes hand in hand with de-stressing, but for a different reason. Listen, infertility is a stressful thing. We totally get it. Many couples rank it as the biggest crisis in their marriage, above things like infidelity and money problems. Couples split up over this stuff. Don't let that be you.

The quest for a baby can consume you if you let it, but you have to choose how it's going to affect you—in a negative way or a positive way. If you let it be negative, then you're going to get depressed every time you get your period, you're going to hate your friends who have babies seemingly just to piss you off, you're going to fight with your spouse because you're just irritable and empty-wombed, and life is generally going to suck. This can go on for years.

But there really, truly is another way to approach this. No matter what happens, stay optimistic and stay open to all possibilities. Don't be so hung up on the one and only way that you want to have a baby that it closes you off to the many other ways you could be happy. Decide up front that if infertility is going to creep into your life, you're going to look at it as an adventure. You may have to work a little harder to get that baby, but how cool is it that one day you're going to have a tangible way to show that kid just how much he was wanted? He was no accident in the back of Daddy's SUV on that night after the playoffs. No! He was so wanted that Mommy and Daddy planned for him and researched and spent all their money and stopped drinking so much and masturbated into a specimen cup and . . . well, maybe the details aren't so important.

You do have some control over this stuff. You can do your part to sort out any problems that may be standing in the way of your fertility, you can do a better job of watching what you eat and drink, and you can get your sexual timing right. If you see that things aren't happening, you can find a fertility doctor with a great track record. Aside from that, it's out of your hands, and you have to accept that your responsibility ends there. Don't let yourself get sucked into a vortex of misery. Decide now that no matter how it all shakes out, you're going to find ways to be happy.

# Part Two

# Infertility

# Chapter 12
# Going to a Fertility Clinic

## Kyra Says . . .

I didn't start out with Jamie. I began the IVF journey at a local clinic, where they put me on high doses of medications to stimulate my ovaries, which seemed to work very well.

"Wow, look at those follicles!" a nurse said during an exam, and I was deeply pleased with myself.

Boy, my life is changing, I thought. Who would have ever thought I would reach a point where a compliment about my follicles would mean so much to me?

Then came my first egg retrieval, where they gave me an anesthetic that acted as a truth serum. I was sufficiently loopy and don't remember the procedure, but I am told that what happened was this:

> **Doctor:** It looks like you have eighteen eggs here! That's amazing. You could be the next Octomom.
> **Me:** Octomom? Fuck that!

I am aware of this conversation only because the nurses were all giggling when I "came to" again, and my husband made me ask

continued on page 192

them what I had said. I was humiliated! "Don't worry—I've heard a lot worse in the operating room," the doctor reassured me. He explained that one of the drugs I'd been given was known to be a "truth serum." Thank goodness they didn't ask me any personal questions; who knows what I might have come out with?

The laughter came to an abrupt end a few days later, however, when not one of those eighteen eggs survived to the embryo stage. The embryologist had combined my eggs with JD's sperm and it just didn't work.

"How are we going to change the protocol next time?" I asked the doctor.

"We're not," he said. "We're just going to try again."

Isn't that the definition of insanity—doing the same thing and expecting different results? I complained to JD that I didn't like the idea of wasting time or money doing the same thing that had already failed, and he mentioned that he knew a terrific fertility doctor through work. He had interviewed a pioneering doctor named Jamie Grifo several times and was impressed by him because of his knowledge and his caring personality.

Jamie was well-respected in the scientific community and had made major strides in preimplantation genetic testing and egg freezing. It was his clinic that first showed that you could get the same success rates from frozen eggs that you could from frozen embryos. The problem was that he was all the way in New York, and we were in Atlanta.

But this is everything, I thought. If ever there was a time to go out of our way and to make the effort to travel, this was it. JD called Jamie, explained our situation and set up an appointment.

What Jamie told me is that my ovaries had been overstimulated and, as a result, they hadn't produced the best-quality eggs.

"So the doctor fried my eggs?" I asked.

"That's a good way to put it," Jamie said. He dialed down my medications, but I still had to stick myself with lots of needles. You learn to get good at it. After about two weeks, I had my second egg retrieval. Again they got eighteen eggs, but this time three of them made it to the blastocyst stage.

When I returned to have the embryos transferred into my uterus, the embryologist put the petri dish under the microscope, flashing my three little blastocysts up on a screen. They were just a circle of cells, but in them I saw the promise of poopy diapers, mashed peas and runny noses. The nurse even printed a picture for us so one day in the future we could show our kid(s) how great things come from the smallest of beginnings. The transfer was a breeze. There was a tiny bit of cramping as Dr. Grifo threaded a skinny catheter through my cervix and into the perfect spot in my uterus. In less than five minutes, the buns were in the oven.

Now we'd just have to wait to see if it worked!

# When to Go to a Clinic

There's no rule about how long you have to wait before going to a clinic. There are guidelines, but it's really up to you. The guideline is that if you're under thirty-five, you're considered infertile if you've been trying for one year without having achieved a pregnancy, or six months if you're thirty-five or older. Don't wait much beyond six months if you're thirty-five or up—your odds will only go down. But you might want to go earlier, if, say, you've had more than one miscarriage, if your periods are extraordinarily painful, if you have pelvic pain or if you have irregular menstrual cycles.

Before going to a fertility clinic, get your FSH score from your OB/GYN. When it comes to IVF, FSH scores are pretty accurate predictors of who's going to be successful and who isn't. It's not as accurate a predictor of unassisted pregnancies, particularly for young women.

Keep in mind that the number of eggs you have is just one part of the story—it doesn't tell you if those eggs are good quality—but it's the important first step. It's smart to have that test done first because it's going to be a very different conversation with a fertility specialist if you know you have a decent number of eggs left as opposed to having very few. A poor ovarian reserve score means there's a very small chance of you getting pregnant with your own eggs, regardless of their quality (though, in general, the fewer eggs left, the poorer the quality). That might also affect whether insurance will cover different treatments. Some insurance plans won't cover fertility treatments for a woman with a poor ovarian reserve as measured by day 3 FSH score. For instance, Aetna defines a poor ovarian reserve as higher than 19 mIU/ml (milli-international units per milliliter), and different Aetna plans handle this in different ways.

## Insurance and Financing

Speaking of insurance, find out early what exactly is covered and what isn't in terms of fertility tests and treatments. Some states require health insurance companies to cover fertility testing and treatments. Fifteen states in the United States have mandated infertility care as of this printing:

| | |
|---|---|
| Arkansas | California |
| Connecticut | Hawaii |
| Illinois | Louisiana |

| | |
|---|---|
| Maryland | Massachusetts |
| Montana | New Jersey |
| New York | Ohio |
| Rhode Island | Texas |
| West Virginia | |

You can visit the National Infertility Association's website at www.resolve.org and look under "Family Building Options" to find out the details of the laws in each of those states, some of which are more generous than others. For instance, in California, group insurers are required to offer some infertility coverage, but not IVF, whereas in Illinois, group insurers and HMOs are required to offer a wide range of services that include up to four egg retrievals (six in a lifetime) and IVF. Depending on your flexibility and finances, if you know you're headed for expensive fertility treatments, you might want to move to one of the states with the best coverage!

There's no getting around it: Without insurance, fertility treatment is expensive. If you have insurance, you likely just have to pay the specialty copayment for your initial testing. Without insurance, you're looking at about $500–$1,000 for the fertility tests. Then it's about $15,000 per cycle of IVF for the medications and the procedures (keeping in mind that it can take several cycles to work).

Even in states without mandated fertility care, though, many insurers do offer some coverage. Shop around and ask specific questions: Which tests and treatments are covered? How many rounds are covered? What are the copayments? Are there lifetime caps? Are there any restrictions based on age or ovarian reserves? Get creative in searching for the right health insurance. Even if you have health insurance through your employer or school, it might pay to buy a policy on your own that will offer you better coverage. You can also call the fertility clinic you plan to use and ask the staff which health insurance plans offer the best coverage.

There are other ways to work things out, too. Some clinics offer payment plans, and you might be able to take out a loan to cover the costs.

You can also visit www.resolve.org for descriptions of fertility financing programs (such as "shared risk" programs, and programs in which you get a refund if you don't get pregnant).

# Your First Clinic Visits

Here's what happens when you go to a fertility clinic for the first time: They ask you a bunch of questions about your medical and surgical history, find out about your ethnic background so they know which genetic tests you'll need, go over your insurance information and make sure you can pay for treatment, look over your medical records and discuss any concerns you have. Usually that first appointment is just for asking questions and going over the procedure, blood tests and maybe an ultrasound to check out your basic anatomy, no freaky medical stuff. You will also meet your reproductive endocrinologist (RE).

The RE will ask you specific personal questions to figure out if you're ovulating, if there are any obvious potential causes of infertility and how you've been trying on your own, such as:

- How long is your menstrual cycle? Is it regular? (Irregular
  cycles could mean that you're not ovulating regularly,
  and short cycles could mean a lack of hormones necessary
  for conception.)

- Are your periods heavy or light? Do you have significant
  cramps? (Checking for signs of endometriosis and
  hormone imbalances.)

- How often do you have unprotected intercourse?
  (Making sure you're "trying enough" on your own.)

- How long have you been trying to conceive?

- Have you had any STDs?

- Have you ever miscarried or terminated a pregnancy?
  (Then you would have "secondary infertility," rather than
  "primary infertility," and each of those outcomes raises
  different potential fertility problems.)

They stick you with needles to take blood for various tests—which is like training for the needle bonanza you're going to have to partake in if you need to have your eggs harvested. At a minimum, they'll check your baseline FSH and LH, if you didn't just have those checked at your OB/GYN, and they will probably test for STDs.

The second appointment is when stuff gets real. You will likely have a test called a hysterosalpingogram to see if your fallopian tubes are blocked.

We want to lie to you and tell you the standard line about how you'll just feel some pressure or some other horse pucky, but we're cursed with a compulsion to tell the truth. The damn test can hurt. But they have to do it because if you have blocked fallopian tubes, then it won't really matter what else you or they do—you're just not going to have a successful pregnancy.

# Blocked Tubes

When one or both of your tubes are blocked, it's called "tubal factor infertility," and it's responsible for about 20 percent of women's infertility. Fallopian tubes are skinny little things, and it's easy for them to get blocked. How? These are the main ways:

- **Pelvic inflammatory disease** (PID).

- **Infections:** Aside from PID, there are many other types of infections that can cause problems with the fallopian tubes. Appendicitis, peritonitis, infections after childbirth, gallbladder infections and inflammatory bowel disease can all cause tubal blockage because of the formation of scar tissue around or at the end of the tubes.

- **Surgeries:** Any kind of surgery near your fallopian tubes can put you at risk for obstructions. Surgery for a past ectopic pregnancy, as well as abortion, removal of ovarian cysts, or other sorts of pelvic surgeries can cause scar tissue that obstructs the fallopian tubes.

- **Structural abnormalities:** Sometimes tubes are just built wrong, usually caused by a birth defect. The tubes may be blocked because there's a "kink" or another anomaly that prevents the egg from traveling properly in and out of the tube.

- **Fibroids.**

- **Endometriosis.**

If the tubes aren't completely blocked, but they are obstructed partially, you're at high risk for ectopic pregnancy—a pregnancy that occurs in the tubes, rather than being able to move freely out into the uterus where the embryo is supposed to grow. Ectopic pregnancies are very dangerous and have to be terminated as quickly as possible. The fertilized egg can't survive anyway, and the mother is at risk of major complications and even bleeding to death. And after surgery to terminate an ectopic pregnancy, you guessed it—you're at even higher risk for blocked tubes and various other fertility problems.

The hysterosalpingogram (also known as HSG) is a standard test where you lie on your back with your feet in those terrific OB/GYN stirrups underneath an X-ray machine. The technician inserts a speculum, just like when you get a Pap smear, and opens it to clear the path to the cervix. Then he cleans the cervix and inserts a tube. The speculum comes out and the dye goes in—contrast dye is sent slowly through the tube to see if it can make the trip through your uterus and fallopian tubes without getting stuck. The technician takes an X-ray to watch the dye as it moves through your body. Ideally, it goes through the fallopian tubes just fine and then just gets absorbed into your body. But the test can cause bad cramping, especially if you are blocked (the dye will cause your fallopian tubes to swell if it can't flow through). It's a good idea to take a pain reliever about an hour before the procedure. Or Klonopin. Or some grain alcohol. Hey, you're not pregnant yet.

Ask a friend to drive you, if possible, just in case the cramps are bad (or in case you took my grain alcohol advice seriously).

It's probably going to hurt for a little while, and then it'll hurt less while the cramping subsides, and then it's not going to hurt anymore and your life will go on and you'll be just dandy and one step closer to pregnant. When you do have a child, you'll find yourself making all kinds of sacrifices and doing uncomfortable things because of love. Some of us just get lucky enough to be able to prove our love early. One day you can tell your child, "I loved you so much before you were even conceived that I had a speculum inserted into my..." On second thought, maybe you'll tell a different story...

A majority of the women who have this test done don't have any significant pain. Some say it's no different than what they feel when they get a normal Pap smear done. Some say it feels like minor menstrual cramps. And one really cool potential side effect is that if you just have a minor blockage, the test itself may fix it.

If you are unfortunate enough to have friends who insist on telling you bad stuff about tests like these, consider it practice for how terrible people are going to be when they tell you their labor stories— like they're trying to win trophies in a Most Awful Labor competition. Close your ears, smile and nod, and don't call these people back until your child is three.

If you are a complete wreck about the test or have had bad reactions to tests like this before, it is possible to be completely sedated for the procedure. Talk to your doctor about it. As our friend Petra can attest, though, the test isn't always a big deal.

*I had talked myself out of doing it. I searched for info about the test online and read some bad comments people made about how painful it was, and how you can get infections afterwards. "Forget it!" I said. I called my doctor's office, spoke to a nurse, and said I was not coming in, period, and she could not make me.*

*She very patiently listened and told me that the vast majority of patients don't have significant pain, and that the chance of infection is tiny. You can't fool me, I thought. I've read the internet.*

*But she kept going on and on about how experienced they were with this sort of test and how necessary it was. I don't know how, but she sort of hypnotized me into agreeing to keep my appointment—if and only if she would literally come in and hold my hand, because she had a really soothing personality. She made good on her promise, leaving whatever she was doing to sit with me and hold my hand during the procedure. The doctor seemed amused, but I told him that this was deadly serious and that if he hurt me, his poor nurse was going to have one very badly squeezed hand.*

*Then I sat back and waited for the world to end. Which it did not. In fact, the whole thing was extremely anticlimactic. I've had pelvic exams that were worse. There was no pain at all, only very minor discomfort for literally about five seconds when they first put the tube in. I didn't feel the dye go through, I didn't have any cramping during or afterwards and I honestly thought they hadn't done the test yet when the doctor said I was done.*

*"That's it?!" I asked. The nurse gave me a hug for my bravery and went off to go talk someone else down from a ledge, I assume. But before she left, she asked me to please go online and tell everyone else to quit worrying about this procedure. I figure this is part of my fulfillment of that promise.*

Even if you know you're going for IVF, which bypasses the fallopian tubes entirely and just puts the embryo straight into the womb, you should get the HSG test anyway to rule out a condition called hydrosalpinx.

Infections can cause the fallopian tubes to get blocked on the end away from the uterus, fill up with fluid and get distended, and having this condition seriously reduces the success rates of IVF. For unknown reasons, you're 50 percent less likely to get pregnant via IVF if you have a hydrosalpinx. There are rarely symptoms (cramping), but usually there are none, and it can be confused with ovarian cysts on an ultrasound.

If you have one or two hydrosalpinges, the doctor will likely advise you to have the tube removed or separated from your uterus. When going through IVF, which is normally expensive, time-consuming and fraught with emotion, you want to know that you're going into it with the best possible chances.

After her first round of tests, Kyra knew that they hadn't found any blockages in her fallopian tubes, they didn't find any STDs or anything structurally wrong, and her ovarian reserves were normal. Essentially, she looked great on paper.

But that doesn't necessarily mean anything. About one-third of infertility is unexplained, or idiopathic. So about one-third of couples who go through a full fertility workup are told they have "idiopathic infertility," which sounds fancy, but is really another way of saying, "We have no idea why you're not getting pregnant. Sorry." So you can pass all the tests with flying colors and still be infertile, because even though fertility science is one of the fastest-growing fields of our generation, it still has some holes to be patched. And because part of getting pregnant is just dumb luck.

A large portion of idiopathic infertility is just age-related fertility decline—no specific reason other than aging eggs and sperm.

# Genetic Testing

Another thing fertility doctors will recommend is that you go for genetic testing before you get pregnant. Genetic screenings have made huge advances recently, and what used to take thousands of dollars and hundreds of needle sticks can now be done with just one blood or saliva test for about $300. It's called the Recombine test and it checks men and women to see if they're carriers of any of 180 genetic diseases. Different ethnic groups are more susceptible for different genetic problems, with Ashkenazi Jews getting screwed the worst. About one in four of them are carriers of a genetic disease. A closed gene pool means a higher incidence of recessive genes in that population.

Here's how genetic testing works: You have forty-six chromosomes, which all come in pairs. You get one of each pair of chromosomes from your mother and one from your father. If both chromosomes in the pair are normal, you're golden. If one is mutated and one is normal, then you're a carrier of that genetic mutation, and if both are abnormal, then you have the disease corresponding to that mutation. So both parents have to be carriers or have the disease in order to pass on a genetic disorder. But if you are a carrier of a genetic disease, you probably wouldn't know because you wouldn't have any symptoms of the disease—and some of the diseases aren't that big a deal, while others . . . are.

Genetic testing can't tell you with 100 percent certainty whether your future babies will have a disease or not, but it can give you a solid idea of the odds. You might find out that, according to your profiles, you'd have a one in four-thousand chance of having a child with cystic fibrosis . . . or a one in four chance. Knowing that people with cystic fibrosis usually don't live past age thirty-six, if you know you have a one in four chance, you then get to think about what to do with that information—do you still want to go through with a pregnancy? Do you want to use an egg or sperm donor? Doctors can't and won't make those decisions for you, but they can help you gain all the information you can ahead of time so you can empower yourself to make the best decisions for your family.

It also can potentially save you from making that decision later— knowing that your baby is at high risk of a certain disease means that if it happens and you find out during your pregnancy, it won't be a shock, and you'll have already thought through whether to continue the pregnancy or terminate it.

## Jamie Says . . .

Most of the time, when a woman learns she's carrying a baby with a serious genetic defect, she decides to terminate the pregnancy. My office is a no-judgment zone: In medical school, I learned to empathize first, judge last—and not judge at all, if possible. So if you decide to keep the baby, we'll be happy for you, and if you decide to terminate, we'll understand and support you. It's important to have a doctor who'll support your decisions, so you may want to cover any particular ethical issues that you feel are important during your first meeting.

Some ethical issues in fertility are trickier than others, such as when a thirty-year-old patient came to see me for egg freezing. The problem? She had active ovarian cancer for the second time and wasn't in treatment yet. The medications to stimulate egg production for the retrieval flood your system with extra estrogen, and cancer feeds on estrogen. Plus, doing the egg retrieval would push back her chemotherapy by another month . . . so no other fertility doctor wanted to work with her. But she kept searching until she came to our clinic, and we understood that this risk was worth it to her. She needed an incentive to keep fighting—and having the possibility of someday thawing out those eggs and making babies with them helped to pull her out of depression. Otherwise, cancer was going to steal a lot more than her hair and her ovaries.

Your relationship with your RE can be very special. He's probably going to see you at a whole range of your most fragile emotions—scared, hopeful, sad, mad and, with any luck . . . overjoyed. A good RE will not only be good at the technicalities of the job, but also be a solid resource for you in navigating your options and your emotions. You're not stuck with the first doctor you see. Speak with a few until you find someone you feel comfortable with.

Ten days after the embryo transfer, I got the call at work to tell me that my blood test was positive: I was pregnant! I was about to go on the air, but I had to step away from my desk for a minute to compose myself and call JD. He let out a whoop on the other end of the phone and yelled, "Oh my God, congratulations, sweetheart! We're pregnant!"

Jamie had told us to take it easy and watch my stress level, so we took a weekend trip to a mountain resort for JD's birthday. The plan was to sleep in, read books by the lake (about parenting, of course), eat yummy food and let those embryos calmly cook.

It was a beautiful fall day. After a long walk and some boating on the fishpond, I headed into one of the warm cabins to get a cup of tea. Life was good. As my chamomile was steeping, the fireplace was going and my husband was racking up the balls on the pool table, I ducked into the bathroom with thoughts about how a baby was going to change our life together. As I dropped my drawers and sat down, I got a shock. There was blood.

I was scared and confused. Was this normal? I had been told that I could "spot" a little bit when the embryos implanted in the uterine wall, but I had a bad feeling. I called Jamie, who told me I needed to get a blood test on Monday first thing. I tried to relax the rest of the afternoon, hoping the bleeding would stop, but it got progressively worse. By the end of the weekend, I was in the full throes of a miscarriage. It was heartbreaking.

continued on page 206

It took a couple of months for me to regroup. Even then, I wasn't sure I wanted to go through it all again. I needed to ready myself physically to take on all the shots, blood tests and emotional challenges again—but I decided to do it. Ten days after the next transfer, I showed a pregnancy, but the hCG numbers were very low. I had what's called a biochemical pregnancy, where the presence of fertilized embryos triggers some hormonal markers but nothing more.

I now had three failures in a row and I was starting to wonder if God was sending me a message. Maybe it wasn't my calling to be a mom. Was I trying to force something that wasn't meant to be? I felt like such a failure and it was getting harder to hold it together at work. I did fine on the air, but behind the scenes I had a lot of moments like Holly Hunter's character in *Broadcast News*.

On the fourth try, Dr. Andy Toledo (who Jamie recommended to monitor me in Atlanta) suggested that I get tested for MTHFR, the genetic mutation where your body does not effectively metabolize folic acid. Sure enough, he was right. We added another shot to my pretransfer regimen—Lovenox, a blood thinner—and Folgard, a pill that contains high-dose folic acid.

Once again, I felt hopeful, but this time, my feelings were tempered by the knowledge that I had been here before, three times. Would this time really be different?

A few days later, I got a sign when we visited my parents in San Diego for the Fourth of July holiday. My dad came out to the patio and told me he had a gift for me. When he handed it to me, I burst out in tears. It was a golf ball that he had found during a recent round. We are avid golfers in our family, and each of us has our own superstitions with regard to which brand of balls to to use. But with this ball, it wasn't the brand that made me cry; it was the personalized message printed on it. In bold red letters, it read: "I'M READY FOR MY NEXT GRANDCHILD." What karma.

From that point on, I took that golf ball with me to every blood test, squeezing it in my left hand as the lab techs stuck me with needles. It was my time. My head was in the right place, my heart felt good and, by God, I had my lucky golf ball!

When it came time for the transfer, we had a difficult decision to make: How many embryos to put in? Jamie surprised us with his recommendation. He suggested the best way to ensure a pregnancy was to transfer all five. Five? Was I ready to become the Quintomom? Or what if none of them took? Then I would have nothing left for another attempt. I was mentally done with the stimulation and egg retrieval process and would rather have needles stuck in my eyes than go through that again. But Jamie was calming in his optimism. Five, he reassured us, was the magic number.

He told me, "If you wait long enough, everything will come to you." Thinking back on his words, I reminded myself that anything worthwhile may require many attempts until the universe says yes. I took a deep breath and made the decision to go for it. I told Jamie to transfer all five embryos.

Ten days later, I got the news. I was pregnant. This time, I had a great hCG level, which indicated a strong normal pregnancy. I exhaled a little and let myself believe that I was going to have a baby.

I wasn't prepared for what came three days later when my hCG levels were tested again. Instead of rising the normal 60 percent, they had more than doubled. Three days after that, they doubled again. Not only was I pregnant, I was really pregnant. Jamie told me there was a good chance I was carrying multiples.

At twenty-one days, we went to the Reproductive Biology Associates office for the first ultrasound. The test is to listen to the fetal heartbeat and determine what the budding fetus and yolk sac look like. In went the vaginal wand that I had grown

continued on page 208

so strangely accustomed to. There it was: a single yolk sac with a tiny little blob inside. The translucent heart was throbbing away. On the ultrasound it made a squishy sort of whooshing sound. So far so good. The nurse wiggled the wand a bit. From behind the first sac appeared another. There were two! She moved the ultrasound again. With my eyes on the monitor, I convulsed so hard I thought I would shoot the wand right out of my vagina and straight through JD's now thumping heart.

I had triplets.

As JD stood there stunned, teary-eyed and full of love, he probably didn't imagine what was going through my mind. I only had two boobs! How would I feed three children?

And then came something else I wasn't expecting: the "talk." The uncomfortable and heart-wrenching discussion about "reduction." In more blatant terms, eliminating a child because of the risk of "high-order multiples."

This is one of the most controversial discussions that take place during fertility treatments. As soon as the subject was broached, I felt sick to my stomach and felt an overwhelming rush of anxiety. My doctors, who had now become friends and close confidants, explained that at my age, trying to carry triplets might endanger the entire pregnancy, even my life. In other words, I could lose everything I had worked so hard for.

We postponed the decision for a week, at which time we went to New York for a visit with Jamie. He noticed that one of the embryos wasn't as strong as the other two; the heart rate was slower and the yolk sac bigger. "I don't think this one is going to make it," he said.

He was right. By the time we did chorionic villus sampling (CVS) to rule out any genetic abnormalities, we found out what was in store for us: We had two completely normal fetuses developing inside my womb. The third embryo had simply faded away. I was relieved, yet sad at the same time.

I won't lie: The process was mentally and physically exhausting. Luckily for me, I had a doctor at the other end of the phone who was patient, reassuring and clear about every step. Even so, I was frustrated and scared. My hope in relaying my story is to prepare you for what might happen, armed with realistic expectations. With the support of a good doctor, you will be better equipped to deal with the stress and disappointments if you don't succeed the first, or like me, the second or third time.

Now we had another big decision to make: names.

# Chapter 13

# Guys and Infertility: Hey, It's Not Just about Us

It turns out that there's this whole other side to infertility that rarely gets talked about. Guys exist! They have sperm! And sometimes it gets screwed up, too!

Age doesn't affect men's fertility as significantly as it affects women's. There is some drop-off, but not much. That's why you see male celebrities becoming dads in their seventies. However, recent research has shown that sperm does age the way eggs do, and can become chromosomally abnormal. It's not as if old 'nads have found the fountain of youth. There is an increased risk for miscarriage as the male ages and, as we already know, that usually means there's a genetic defect in the embryo. So it's not all that surprising to find out that aging sperm is linked with increased risk for autism, Down syndrome and other genetic abnormalities. A 2012 study in the journal *Nature* showed that there's a directly correlated risk as a man ages that his child will have autism or schizophrenia, unrelated to the age of the mother.[1]

De novo mutations are new alterations in a gene as a result of a mutation in an egg or sperm cell or the fertilized egg. The study showed that babies inherited, on average, fifteen de novo genetic mutations from the mother, but the number of mutations they inherited from the father increased with every year of the father's age. So a baby fathered by a twenty-year-old man had, on average, twenty-five de novo mutations from his father, and that number increased by two mutations for every year of the father's age, until there were sixty-five mutations for babies fathered by men who were forty. The researchers estimate that up to 30 percent of autism cases may be linked to these de novo mutations.

One of the things that pisses us off about the way our society views fertility is that it's a "woman thing." Often, men don't even bother getting tested until after the woman does, because they assume that infertility is the woman's fault. Women then bear the brunt of the blame and guilt for infertility. Neither sex should feel guilty about infertility. Guilt is for suckers. But when we get down to causes, don't assume that the lion's share of fertility rests on a woman's shoulders . . . or ovaries.

Even though it's true that age doesn't have the same effect on a man's fertility, that doesn't mean that they're all delivering SuperSperm. In fact, in the cases where the cause of infertility is known, it's caused by the male's sperm just as often as it's caused by the female's eggs—about 30–40 percent of infertility is caused by male factors, 30–40 percent by female factors, many cases by both, and the rest are unknown. There may be several reasons for male-factor infertility.

For a man to be fertile, several things need to happen: He needs to have enough sperm to make the journey to the egg, they need to travel fast enough and have enough strength to penetrate the egg, and they have to be shaped correctly and contain the proper genetic material. Here's what could go wrong:

- **AZOOSPERMIA:** That's when there's no measurable level of sperm in the man's semen. It's not that he's not ejaculating—he is—but he's "shooting blanks." That could be because of a wide variety of things, including genetic abnormalities in his testes, environmental factors, injury or use of certain substances or medications (or, of course, if he's had a vasectomy). You wouldn't notice anything wrong in a normal sexual situation because only a tiny percentage (less than 5 percent) of semen is actually sperm cells. Most of it is fluid from places other than the testicles—proteins and sugars, primarily. So if you've ever had a guy try to convince you that semen is good for you because it's high in protein . . . well, he's kind of right. Each ejaculate has about as much protein as an egg white. About 6 percent of infertile men have some kind of obstruction that's causing azoospermia (which can sometimes be fixed by surgery), and about 15 percent of infertile men have azoospermia that's not related to any kind of obstruction.

- **OLIGOZOOSPERMIA:** When there are sperm present, but in lower-than-normal levels, it's called oligozoospermia. That's the case in about 65 percent of infertile men. It may also be accompanied by other sperm problems.

- **ASTHENOZOOSPERMIA:** This refers to sperm with reduced motility. The sperm might not be fast enough, or they may swim crooked or not really move at all—just swishing their tails around, kind of like treading water. Normally, at least half of sperm should have good motility.

- **TERATOZOOSPERMIA:** This refers to sperm with abnormal shapes. *Terato* comes from the Greek word for "monster," so, yeah. Monster sperm. And it's totally normal for a large proportion of sperm cells to be imperfect, but at least 15 percent of them have to be right or else it's considered teratozoospermia. The sperm may have two heads, no tail, a round head instead of an oval head, a head that's too tiny or too big or any other abnormality that prevents it from doing its job and fertilizing the egg.

- **OLIGOASTHENOTERATOZOOSPERMIA:** That's the mouthful of a word they use when all three of the main factors are present—low sperm count, reduced motility and high numbers of abnormally shaped sperm.

- **SPERM ANTIBODIES:** Our bodies normally produce antibodies to fight off threats such as bacterial infections. But every now and then, our bodies get confused and see something normal as an invader. Some men produce antibodies that kill their own sperm. This can happen after a vasectomy and persist even if the vasectomy is reversed. It can also happen in cases of infections, and for unknown reasons.

# Preventable Causes of Male Infertility

Just as with female infertility, some things are within your control and some aren't. There are genetic defects that cause infertility, as well as unavoidable damage done by things like cancer and cancer treatments. But there are also things men can do to screw up their fertility:

- **ANABOLIC STEROID USE:** Prolonged use of steroids can cause azoospermia, a reduction in sperm cells and abnormal sperm cells. "Stacking" steroids (using more than one kind at a time) increases the problem. Normally, sperm production goes back to normal after the guy has stopped using steroids for a few months. Meanwhile, even though steroids often make guys hornier, it's like a cruel joke because it negatively affects their ability to get an erection. Which is obviously bad for babymaking, too.

- **ALCOHOLISM:** Heavy drinking (averaging more than six drinks a day) can hinder the quantity and quality of sperm.

- **SMOKING:** Smoking decreases sperm count.

- **SEXUALLY TRANSMITTED DISEASES:** Just as in women, STDs in men also play a major factor in infertility. Chlamydia, gonorrhea and herpes have all been proven to negatively affect sperm production.

- **DRUGS:** Regular use of marijuana can lower sperm count, cause poor sperm motility and reduce the volume of seminal fluid. Other drugs, such as cocaine, methamphetamine, heroin and ecstasy, can cause low sperm counts and abnormally shaped sperm. It's not known how long these effects last after someone has stopped using the drugs, but it seems to be a problem when the drug use is frequent, not when someone has just "experimented" a few times. So if there were a few times in college...you're probably fine. Long-term opiate use can lower testosterone and cause male infertility—this applies to both prescription opiates (painkillers) and street drugs.

- **HIGH BMI:** When men get chunky, their sperm get lazy. A BMI over 25 puts them at higher risk of having problems with sperm's shape and motility.

- **OVERHEATED TESTICLES:** Anything that causes the testicles to heat up even one degree past normal body temperature can temporarily halt or slow down sperm production. That includes things like saunas and hot tubs. Wearing boxers instead of tighty whiteys is a good idea, though unlikely to make a big difference. But sperm counts are typically higher in winter and lower in summer, which is probably because of temperatures "in the sack." Get it? In the sack? Hooray for puns!

- **HIGH BLOOD PRESSURE:** It's not really the condition itself that causes fertility problems but the medications. They can cause problems with erections and ejaculation, including retrograde ejaculation (see next section). So if you can help him regulate his high blood pressure naturally, then do it! Get him into better diet and exercise routines and see if you can lessen or eliminate the need for medication.

- **SLEEP APNEA:** It's hard to decide whether to put this one in the "preventable" or "out of your control" category, because it can go either way. Sleep apnea is a condition where you wake up several times a night because you've temporarily stopped breathing. You typically don't remember waking up, but your body does, in fact, go all conscious for a second because you stopped breathing. Jeez. It's caused by blocked or narrowed airways in your throat, mouth or nose. Most often, sleep apnea is a product of being overweight or obese, but it can also be caused by a large uvula, tonsils or adenoids. It's most common in men who sleep on their backs, and they're typically loud snorers. It's worse for guys who drink or take certain medicines before bed. If you sleep next to someone with sleep apnea, you may hear a whole symphony of disturbing noises—snoring, choking, gasping. And it can lead to chronic sleep deprivation, even if he thinks he's slept all night. He never really gets enough deep sleep because his sleep keeps getting interrupted, which leads to a bunch of problems: depression, anxiety, moodiness, high blood pressure . . . and infertility.

- **HIGH PROLACTIN LEVELS:** A few small studies have shown that men who were treated with CPAP (continuous positive airway pressure) machines improved their prolactin levels. You want low prolactin levels; high levels interfere with the production of testosterone and lower the sex drive.

- **OBESITY:** Whether or not he has sleep apnea, being obese can significantly affect a man's testosterone levels and ability to get an erection, as well as messing up his sperm quality and quantity.

- **DISTURBED SLEEP:** Not only because of sleep apnea, but any kind of sleep disturbances can throw off both male and female fertility. A new study from Denmark showed that men who had the most disturbed sleep (trouble falling asleep, trouble staying asleep) also had the lowest sperm counts: 29 percent lower than average, and less normal-shaped sperm as well.[2]

# Causes of Male Infertility That Are, More or Less, Out of Your Control

There are many causes of male infertility that are not usually caused by our conscious decisions. Some have temporary effects and some have permanent effects.

- **FEVER:** Getting the flu, or any other illness that involves a high fever, can temporarily mess up sperm or even cause temporary azoospermia. Sperm typically return to normal levels within four to six months. Before that period is over, you can still get pregnant, but sperm is not at optimal levels.

- **MUMPS:** Mumps, on the other hand, can permanently mess up sperm. Not only does it cause fever, but it also causes swelling and inflammation in the testicles, called mumps orchitis, which can result in sterility because sperm production is permanently halted.

- **VARIOCELES:** The most common physical cause of male infertility is varioceles—enlarged veins in the scrotum, like varicose veins in the legs. They're usually easy to detect because the scrotum looks like—and forgive me for how gross this is— a bag of worms. About 10 percent of all men have varioceles, and 30 percent of infertile men have them. Varioceles almost always occur on the left side and can hinder sperm count and quality and can even cause the testicles to shrink. This condition is treatable by surgery or embolization (creating a blockage in the veins), but that doesn't always bring fertility levels up to normal. Repair of large varioceles shows a greater improvement in fertility than repair of smaller varioceles.

- **UNDESCENDED TESTICLES:** A boy's testicles normally descend from the abdomen into the scrotum before birth; if one or both of them don't, it's called undescended testicles. Doctors usually perform surgery when the testicles don't descend by age one, but even once the problem is fixed, it still raises the risk of infertility down the line.

- **EXPOSURE TO ENVIRONMENTAL HAZARDS:** As they do with women, environmental hazards, such as pesticides, paint, lead and solvents, affect fertility in different ways. Working or living in a hazardous environment that exposes you to radiation or toxic chemicals can have a serious impact on male fertility and miscarriage rates.

- **HORMONE PROBLEMS:** Low testosterone and other hormonal deficiencies can hinder fertility.

- **CELIAC DISEASE:** The digestive disorder celiac disease can harm male fertility, and there's some proof that adopting a gluten-free diet can help reverse this.

- **POLYCYSTIC KIDNEY DISEASE:** The cysts can block sperm production.

- **RETROGRADE EJACULATION:** This occurs when some or all of the semen goes "backwards" into the bladder rather than out through the urethral tip. This usually happens because the bladder neck fails to close. It can also be caused by diabetes, medications used to treat hypertension, and medications or surgery to treat prostate or urethra problems. If it's caused by a medication, then stopping that medication will usually solve the problem, but if it's a structural problem or caused by diabetes, it's usually not fixable. However, a doctor can still retrieve the sperm and use it in IVF.

- **INJURIES TO GENITALS:** Remember when you were watching that Little League game and a kid threw his bat and accidentally smashed another kid in the nuts, and someone said, "Oooh, there goes his chances of having kids"? And then people sort of winced and giggled? Well, it could be true. Maybe. Those damn testicles can rupture! Even seemingly minor injuries from sports or trauma can have long-standing effects on a man's ability to get an erection and his fertility.

Surgery performed right after the injury can help to save the testicle.

- **Spinal cord injury:** Depending on the specifics of the injury, spinal cord injuries often have a major effect on a man's fertility (and a minor effect, if any, when it happens to a woman). In many cases, men are unable to ejaculate normally afterwards. This doesn't mean that men with spinal cord injuries can't father children, however—it just means that interventions may be needed. There are techniques a couple can try at home, and others that need to be done in a fertility lab.

- **Klinefelter's syndrome:** Most men with Klinefelter's syndrome have one extra copy of the X chromosome in each cell. This can lead to a variety of physical and psychological symptoms, including small testes, low testosterone, reduced facial hair, breast enlargement and irreversible infertility.

Finding out that your partner has a fertility problem can put strain on the relationship. Suddenly you're mad at him for his crooked-swimming monster sperm and thinking through all the ways he may have caused this by being irresponsible and falling off a motorcycle or messing around with cocaine ten years ago or getting an STD or doing something so stupid that made that girl want to kick him in the groin and rupture his sack. Or maybe there's no discernible reason at all and you're still just mad at him for not somehow whipping those sperm into shape. Like, couldn't he just try a little harder? Sheesh.

And because men usually assume that infertility is the woman's fault, finding out that they have a problem can cause a lot of anger, guilt and self-esteem issues. You know how some men announce, "My boys can swim!" when their partner gets pregnant? The flip side of that macho brag, "My boys are slow and shaped funny," is not a fun thing for a guy to acknowledge.

But it's something to prepare for when you go in for testing—if you get any answers as to why you're not getting pregnant, they may be factors related to you, your partner or both of you, and you can't let that undermine your relationship. You both have to go into it knowing that no matter how the tests turn out, there's no one to blame, just a team working together to make the best decisions you can with whatever information you get.

# Vitamins and Supplements That Can Boost Men's Fertility

It takes about three months for sperm to develop and mature, so that's how long it'll take to see any appreciable difference after making lifestyle changes and adding vitamins and supplements to his routine.

- **FOLIC ACID:** Usually thought of as a women's supplement, we now know that folic acid is good for men, too. In one study, men who took the highest levels of folate and folic acid in their diet and in supplement form—between 722 and 1,150 micrograms per day—had a 20–30 percent reduction in chromosomally abnormal sperm.[3]

- **VITAMIN C:** Vitamin C improves sperm in every way. Studies have shown that taking vitamin C supplements daily can improve sperm count, motility and shape. Aim for at least 1,000 mg per day.

- **VITAMIN D:** Vitamin D is the "sunshine vitamin," and infertile men are getting too little of it. Sperm has a vitamin

D receptor, and it turns out that at least 25 percent of men who are infertile have lower than normal levels of vitamin D. Just as with vitamin C, adding vitamin D supplements can improve sperm in every way. The recommended daily intake for an adult male is 600 IU (or 15 mcg).

- **Zinc:** Zinc sulfate helps with sperm morphology (shape), in particular, and can improve the outcome after surgery for variocele repair. Aim for 100–200 mg per day in food or supplement form. Researchers have found major benefits by combining zinc sulfate and folic acid supplementation in men with fertility problems.

- **Coenzyme Q10 (CoQ10):** Several studies have now shown that treating men who have fertility problems with CoQ10 supplements improves sperm count and motility. He can take 100–300 mg in two divided doses each day to keep the levels up in the bloodstream.

- **Royal Jelly:** Royal Jelly is a secretion of worker honey bees, and it's rich in amino acids. It's the exclusive food given to the queen bee to help her lay eggs. One relatively small study showed that infertile men who were given 25–100 mg of Royal Jelly a day increased their sperm's motility, as well as their testosterone levels and libido.[4] However, it can cause an allergic reaction if you're allergic to pollen.

# Chapter 14:
# I Have to Put That Needle Where?

Depending on the cause of your infertility, your age, budget and other factors, there are several fertility treatment options that you might use.

## Fertility Drugs

If the problem has to do with your ovulation or his sperm quality, your doctor may just try putting you on medications to see if you conceive naturally after that. It's the cheapest and least invasive option. Cost varies, depending on whether you take pills (much cheaper) or injections (costlier, but more effective).

## Intrauterine Insemination

Intrauterine insemination (IUI) is a fairly simple procedure in which a doctor washes sperm to separate motile sperm from seminal fluid, then injects it right into the woman's uterus—saving it the trip. It's also known as artificial insemination and is the most common fertility treatment. It's an appropriate option in any of these situations:

- Low sperm count
- Low sperm motility
- Unexplained infertility
- Hostile cervical environment, such as thick or acidic mucus
- Woman has developed antibodies to the man's sperm
- When using donor sperm

You may be encouraged to take fertility medications, such as Clomid, before the procedure so that you have the chance of maturing more than one follicle, and thus having more than one chance of getting pregnant per cycle. The procedure itself shouldn't be painful and you won't need anesthesia. It's just a thin, flexible tube that gets inserted and it's a quick outpatient procedure.

Success rates are about 10–15 percent per cycle, and a doctor may want you to try at least two to three IUI cycles before moving on. Know up front how many cycles he wants you to do and what the next step would be if it's not successful, and make sure that matches up with what you think is reasonable for your own time line and budget. If you're pushing the edge of your fertility, you might want to just try one or two IUI cycles and not more than that, whereas you might want to try more if you're younger. Aside from the cost of medications (which can vary a lot), the procedure itself costs about $865 per cycle, according to the National Infertility Association RESOLVE. However, they note that that figure is variable because some clinics include bloodwork, medication and ultrasounds in their pricing while others don't. Make sure to clarify what's included if you're comparison shopping.

# The IVF Procedure

IVF (in vitro fertilization) is when sperm is combined with an egg in a dish. It may become fertilized on its own in there, or the doctor may use

ICSI (intracytoplasmic sperm injection) to inject one sperm right into the middle of the egg cell. In certain situations, such as when eggs have been frozen, ICSI is necessary. It adds about $1,500–$2,500 to the cost.

After an egg is fertilized, it begins to divide and becomes an embryo. Doctors will try to make as many embryos as they can, and then somewhere between day 3 and day 5, transfer them back into the woman's uterus.

## What the Patient Goes Through

IVF has several steps. First, you need to get checked out to make sure that you're a good candidate and that your body can handle a pregnancy. Once you're cleared for takeoff, you come into the clinic on day 2 of your cycle to get an ultrasound (we know … an ultrasound on your period … ick) and a blood test to check on your estrogen levels. Provided the doctor says you're ready, you then start injecting yourself with fertility drugs—usually gonadotropins, including Repronex, Follistim, Gonal F, and Menopur. They are to help you develop more than one mature egg this cycle.

On cycle day 7 to 9, you'll begin taking another medication: a GnRH agonist, meant to block the release of luteinizing hormone (which would cause you to ovulate). Finally, when the doctor deems that your follicles are ready, you'll take the final shot: hCG, which mimics the LH surge and fully matures your eggs. In some cases, a doctor will prescribe a shot of Lupron instead of hCG to mature the eggs. You have to take it at a very exact time, because thirty-five hours later, you'll have your egg retrieval.

If you're using frozen or donor sperm, it'll already be in the lab. If not, then on the same day as your egg retrieval, your partner will provide the sperm either at the clinic or in a specimen cup from home. It's kind of unfair that the only pain he has to go through in all of this is that he has to take antibiotics before giving his sperm sample (to minimize risk of infection to the embryo). Well, that and dealing with your potential mood swings and complaining about the effects of the medications! It's true—the medications can cause all sorts of hormonal reactions and discomfort. Some women have very slight side effects and others feel like they're on emotional roller coasters.

Michelle was one of the roller-coaster girls.

*My emotional reaction started even before I began the medications. I hated the thought of going through IVF. It made me angry that we weren't able to get pregnant on our own. I was young and healthy and so was my husband, and I thought the universe owed us a baby. Worse, it seemed that everyone I knew was having babies all at once while we were going through infertility, and my best friend got pregnant on her first try twice.*

*I cried every time I went to the clinic. Every time. I couldn't go to another baby shower or kid's birthday party. I was just so hurt.*

*I also cried the first time I saw the giant bag of medication from the pharmacy. It was like a physical reminder of the "unnaturalness" of it all. The staff at my clinic couldn't have been nicer about it all, and my boss was very understanding when I explained that I'd have to come in late several days due to doctor's appointments, but I still felt miserable. We had already failed at a medication-only approach and three rounds of IUI, so this was our next option.*

*The fact that I was already depressed did not mix well with the hormonal party caused by the medications. I was mad at my husband for no good reason even as I made him do my injections. I just wanted to sleep and cry most of the time.*

*One thing that helped was to schedule some "good touch" time to counteract the fact that I was feeling so poked and prodded all the time. I got a massage, manicure and pedicure. It made me remember that my body wasn't just a science experiment.*

*And then . . . the positive pregnancy test.*

*My son is now seven months old.*

*I'm not sure if I've stopped smiling since.*

*We have several frozen embryos waiting for us now, and I've helped counsel friends who have started the fertility journey. It wasn't the way I ever imagined having a baby, but believe me when I say that this little boy doesn't feel "unnatural" to me in any way. He's ours and he's wonderful. Science is good.*

# Donor Eggs, Donor Sperm and Surrogacy

Women rarely want to consider the possibility of using donor eggs, but it is one way to still have a pregnancy and have some control over those nine months in a way that adoption and surrogacy don't provide.

When considering the issue of donor sperm, one important ethical and practical concern has come up in the media in recent years: Some clinics allow the same donor to father dozens, or even upwards of a hundred children. That can be disturbing when you consider that the donor's children likely live in the same geographic area and can run into each other . . . incest may happen unintentionally, and so may the propagation of genetic disorders. There are now limits in Great Britain: Each donor may father no more than ten children. But there are no such limits in the United States yet, only guidelines. Ask your clinic if they impose any limits on donors.

You may also choose to use a surrogate—either someone you know or someone you hire for this purpose. The surrogate may use your egg and your partner's sperm, her own egg and your partner's sperm, her egg and donor sperm . . . there are several possible permutations.

## What Will You Deal with Emotionally?

Potentially, a lot. Surveys have shown that fertility patients are just as depressed as cancer patients. Even though fertility is not a mortality issue, it's a major quality of life issue—if you want to have a baby and you can't, then a significant part of you feels "missing" and is not easy to replace.

For many, every negative pregnancy test is a major loss. It's another month that they "failed." Women often start looking at time as their enemy, and days don't really matter except for that one day of truth each month: testing day.

It would ring hollow for either of us to tell you not to let it get to you like that. But Jamie hopes that women will not see themselves as victims. We grow up thinking that it's our natural right to have babies when we want to, and that's just not true. Not all women can have biologically related babies, even with IVF. Of course that's a terrible thing to find out and accept, but for some of us, it will be true, and then you have to figure out a way to move on—either by finding another way to have a child in your life or to decide to remain child-free.

But assuming that you are still a candidate for IVF, know that you may feel like you're at war for a while. You'll have to give yourself injections at least twice a day at regular times, no matter where you are. You'll have to spend a lot of time in the fertility clinic, sometimes getting poked and prodded. Your surging hormones may cause all sorts of emotional reactions—moodiness, anger, changes to your sex drive and so on—and you may start noticing all the pregnant women around you and kind of hating them.

Ideally, your IVF will be successful quickly and these feelings will go away. But know that you may be in for a marathon instead of a sprint. As much as you can, find ways to do things that take your focus off fertility during this process. Go to the movies, exercise, talk to friends, go dancing, read a book, paint a picture. Keep yourself busy and fire up those endorphins in your brain.

## Kyra Says . . .

Okay, so I told you that I had a hemorrhoid story. You've waited long enough to hear it.

You may or may not know that lots of pregnant women get hemorrhoids. You can get them during pregnancy, and you can also get them while you're pushing out that bowling ball of a baby if you have a vaginal birth. But you probably don't know that all the medications you take during fertility treatment can also make you very constipated, which can lead to . . . yep, you guessed it. The big "H." Jamie warned me about it and told me to eat a high-fiber diet and drink lots of water so I wouldn't get constipated, but I was convinced that this kind of thing would never happen to me.

So there I was on a business trip when the darn thing popped out. It was awful. My mom called all the little old ladies at church to get a recommendation to the best butt doctor around. I figured it would be a discreet sort of thing, visiting a doctor who specializes in removing hemorrhoids, but instead, there was the sign outside in unmistakable letters: SAN DIEGO COLON & RECTAL CENTER. I hoped there were no photographers around.

The first thing I saw was a giant stuffed animal mounted on the wall, and thought that was a cute thing for a doctor's office . . . except that it was a polar bear's backside, with one leg lifted in the air. Where most waiting rooms have the latest magazines, this one had only butt books: *The Gas We Pass, Everybody Poops,* and so on. Everyone in the room was smirking.

The doctor's first words to me were, "Drop your pants and let's take a look at your little friends."

I did as I was told and she said, "Oh, that's a problem."

So while I was staring straight ahead at a framed T-shirt of a person with a daisy growing out of his butt and the caption "Yup, too much fiber," the doctor set about the business of taping my butt cheeks wide open to either side of the table.

"Wow, honey, I've never seen you like this before," my dear JD said.

Women may freak you out with their childbirth stories, but I'm here to say this: Needles in your butt are exactly as unpleasant as you'd imagine. Listen to your doctor. Load up on fiber and stay regular. You so don't want to end up on the wrong side of the table at a rectal center.

# People Say Stupid Things

One thing that you should prepare yourself for is the very distinct possibility that someone, somewhere is going to say deeply hurtful things about the choices you've made. For Michelle, that came in the form of a good friend's father—a man she has a great relationship with. His religion, however, doesn't support IVF. When she announced her pregnancy, he wasn't as congratulatory as she expected.

"I just think that if it's not meant to be, it's not meant to be and you shouldn't try to change God's will," he told her. He said that he would have understood if she'd wanted to adopt, but he didn't agree with their decision to go for IVF. "I'll support you anyway," he added.

Gee, thanks, she didn't say. It was hurtful to her that he wanted to impose his belief system on her and that he was trying to make her feel guilty for the life growing inside her.

There are some religions that oppose IVF but don't oppose certain subsets of it, namely GIFT (gamete intrafallopian transfer) and ZIFT (zygote intrafallopian transfer). Those are rare procedures that begin the same way as IVF—with egg harvesting and mixing with sperm in a petri dish—but with GIFT, the egg-and-sperm mix is then just put directly into the fallopian tubes so that fertilization can happen naturally in the body. With ZIFT, the fertilized eggs (called zygotes) are transferred into the fallopian tubes within twenty-four hours, before they become embryos. However, these procedures require an extra surgery and are more expensive than IVF. They also don't allow "Darwin in the lab": embryologists who can see which embryos remain viable after three to five days. That's why IVF is used in 98 percent of cases and ZIFT and GIFT are used in only 2 percent.

In addition to religious concerns, people may just make insensitive remarks about how you should give up or that it's "not natural" or that there are plenty of babies out there who need adoption. This is part of the reason why there's a stigma about IVF that's hard to overcome; not everyone "gets it." Not everyone will be supportive in the way that you'd hope. Focus on the people who are, and hope the others come around. That's the best you can do.

# You Can Still Get Postpartum Depression

It's a funny thing—people sometimes think that you get postpartum depression because you're not really happy about becoming a mother. But in cases where IVF has been used, you know that the person is pretty darn committed to becoming a mother; not only has she tried to have a baby, but she's also spent a lot of time and money on it and stuck needles all over her body and withstood medical tests and interventions in order to make it happen. Quite possibly, she's done it more than once and has even likely been through the trauma of miscarriage. Still, she persists because she wants a baby that much.

Why, then, would she get depressed when the very thing she's been hoping for shows up in her life?

Depression isn't a logical thing. Postpartum depression is a common occurrence—when it's mild, they call it the "baby blues" (which usually lasts just a week or so), but when it persists or gets extreme, then it gets its official classification. The exact reasons for this phenomenon aren't known, but it's very likely that hormones play a major role. Your body is a giant bag full of hormones during pregnancy, and they drop off sharply right after labor. Estrogen and progesterone levels go way down within hours.

Combine that with the exhaustion you likely feel and the sleep deprivation that's a rite of passage for new parents, the understandable fears and anxieties about how to care for a newborn, and the physical changes you're adjusting to, and you have a perfect setup for your brain to go a little out of whack.

So let me reiterate: It can happen no matter how much you want your baby. It can happen to anyone. We're lucky that women are starting to talk about this and normalize it. Celebrities such as Brooke Shields,

Gwyneth Paltrow, Amanda Peet, Courteney Cox and Lisa Rinna have all written about it or talked about it in interviews.

## Kyra Says . . .

Guess what? Now I lend my voice to the chorus: Yes, it happened to me, too—I didn't expect it and didn't know how to deal with it at first, but I felt overwhelmed and antisocial. I found myself pacing around the house for hours and I didn't want anyone around for the first few months after the twins were born. I snapped at JD and worried that things would never feel good again.

JD insisted that I see a doctor, which just made me angry. When the doctor asked why I was there, I said, "I don't know. Ask HIM. He made me come here!" Then I burst into tears. That might have given the doctor a clue!

It lasted for about three months, and I was able to beat it by attacking the problem from several angles, such as cutting out caffeine and alcohol, getting exercise, getting out of the house by myself sometimes and taking an anti-anxiety medication before bed only when needed.

You're more prone to postpartum depression if you've ever experienced depression or other mental health problems before, if you don't have a good support system in place, if you get less than six hours sleep a night, if you're having relationship problems or if you have physical problems after the birth. But lots of times, there is no identifiable cause. It just happens, and there is no shame in it. There is help available, and you won't feel bad forever. Eventually, it'll get good, and then awesome. When people say they never knew how much love they could feel before they became parents? Totally true.

## Chapter 15
# Recent Developments in Fertility Treatments

The first "test-tube baby" was born in 1978 in England, taking a major step forward in the practice of fertility science. In the decades since, we've seen great strides in technology and in our knowledge base to treat infertility. Here are some of the latest developments that you may not know about yet.

## Preimplantation Genetic Screening

Preimplantation genetic screening (PGS), also known as preimplantation genetic diagnosis (PGD) is an exciting new development that has radically changed fertility care. Now doctors can get an egg and sperm together, wait a few days to see if they begin to make an embryo and then test it to see if it's chromosomally normal. If it isn't, it doesn't get implanted, thus lowering the risk of an unsuccessful IVF cycle, miscarriage or a baby being born with Down syndrome.

Without any kind of screening, the risk for miscarriage is high in IVF (over 40 percent for women over forty, and as high as 15–20 percent for women under thirty) because so many genetically abnormal embryos are implanted, most of which wouldn't have resulted in a pregnancy from sex.

That's important to fertility professionals because we know that a miscarriage is not just like a seed that didn't develop; it's a death in the family. Seeing how devastated women are after a miscarriage is one of the toughest parts of Jamie's job, so he'd rather do the screenings and implant fewer embryos than put women and couples through that kind of trauma.

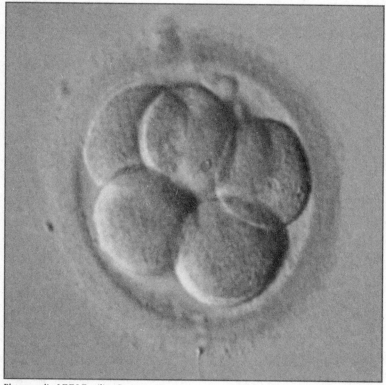

Photo credit: NYU Fertility Center

Day 3 embryo consisting of eight cells

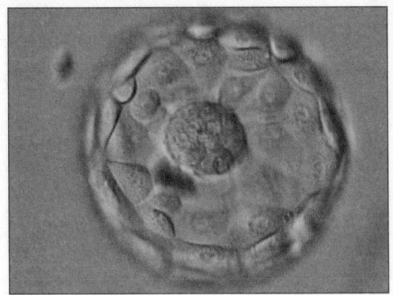

Photo credit: NYU Fertility Center
Day 5 blastocyst

## Trophectoderm Biopsy

Trophectoderm biopsy has given fertility doctors a new window on embryos so they can tell what's going on before they decide which ones—and how many—to implant. In 1990, they had the first professional meeting about PGD and the doctors all left there fired up with the knowledge that, someday, they were going to be able to test embryos and check all the chromosomes.

In the beginning of genetic testing in 1992, Jamie's team would wait for day 3 of an embryo's development. The embryo would have just a few cells at that point, and they'd remove one cell for testing. The tests were limited; they couldn't check all the chromosomes, but they could test five to nine chromosomes to see if they were normal. Another problem was what's known as mosaicism: Not all cells in an embryo are necessarily the same. Sometimes there are DNA mutations

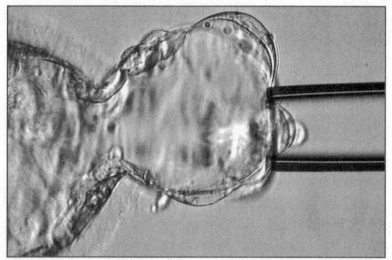

Photo credit: NYU Fertility Center

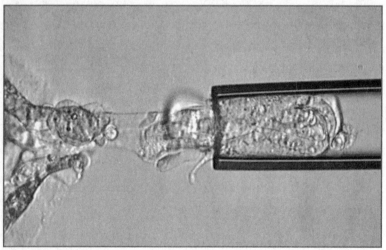

Photo credit: NYU Fertility Center
Day 5 trophectoderm biopsy

or errors. Finally, taking one cell out of an eight-cell embryo was a lot—those embryos could still result in healthy pregnancies, but there was the concern of damaging the embryo by removing a cell for testing.

This type of genetic testing did help to filter out some chromosomally abnormal embryos, but it wasn't enough information and it was an imperfect system.

Now they use a much better, more specialized technique once the embryo hits the blastocyst stage. Normally, that happens on day 5, after the egg is combined with the sperm.

Prior to this type of screening, it was rare for fertility doctors to wait five days before implanting the embryos into the woman—three or four days was the norm (and in many practices, still is). But waiting until the blastocyst stage means that you can start seeing which cells are going to become part of the fetus and which ones will become the placenta and membrane. Then you can take a few of the placenta and membrane cells and analyze them to screen for genetic defects. It's less risky to the embryo, not susceptible to mosaicism, and much more accurate. In fact, so far, Jamie has had less than a 1 percent error rate using this method. In one instance, a woman miscarried after this screening and a biopsy revealed that the embryo was genetically abnormal. This was the only false negative result he's had thus far.

The other advantage to waiting until the blastocyst stage is that it allows "Darwin in the lab" to work. Charles Darwin wrote about natural selection—or survival of the fittest. When doctors implant embryos on day 3, they don't find out which ones nature is going to take care of on its own—some of those embryos that looked fine to a trained eye won't make it to blastocysts because they're not strong enough or genetically sound. On day 5, some chromosomally abnormal embryos remain, which is why testing is still important.

It took twenty years after that first meeting for the technology and techniques to be advanced enough to use them in normal clinical practice. This is what Jamie's team found:

## Chromosomally Normal Chart

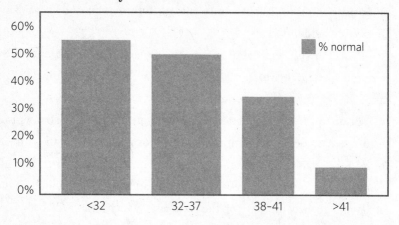

When they analyzed embryos from women under age thirty-two, 53 percent were chromosomally normal and at least theoretically capable of making healthy babies. (Some normal embryos still don't result in a pregnancy, much in the same way that you typically have to plant several seeds in the ground to get one healthy plant.) However, in women over the age of forty-one, just 10 percent of the embryos were normal. Of the remaining 90 percent, very few of them would go on to make babies if implanted—and if they did survive, a large portion would be chromosomally abnormal and unhealthy.

Using trophectoderm biopsy has changed a ton about the way fertility doctors can do their jobs, and it's made for major advances in the field since 2010. As a result of waiting until the blastocyst stage and testing embryos, miscarriage rates have been significantly cut in IVF, and doctors can put back one embryo at a time because they know which ones are "good" embryos, rather than implanting two or more and hoping for the best. So the testing also means that there are now fewer twins, triplets and beyond due to IVF methods—and conversely, a much better chance of a successful singleton pregnancy.

Jamie would like to see all of his patients use preimplantation genetic screening, but many don't because of the cost—it adds $6,000 to the bill. But if you consider the added costs of care for multiple births, stays in the neonatal intensive care unit, termination of a pregnancy if it's found that a fetus has serious genetic problems and so on, he says that, on average, it's cheaper to screen.

Aside from cost, about the only downside is that sometimes there are no genetically perfect blastocysts. In fact, sometimes there are no blastocysts at all because they die off before that point. Of course, that leads to a lot of disappointment for the women and couples who just went through the effort and cost of IVF for nothing... but it also saves them the greater heartache of a failed pregnancy or the difficult decision about what to do if a fetus is found to have significant problems. It can also help people move to the next step if they have the information that all of the embryos were chromosomally abnormal; whereas before they might have just kept trying and trying because no one could explain why they weren't getting pregnant. Knowing that they're just not producing healthy embryos could help a woman or couple make the decision to try another method of having a baby (such as egg donor or adoption).

# Choosing Your Baby's Sex

The ethics of this are entirely up to you to decide, but it is possible now, using PGD, to know whether an embryo is male or female. It's not the same test that screens for genetic abnormalities, but is part of that same type of testing. You can choose the sex of your baby based on this. Both fertile and infertile couples have used this type of testing; sometimes, a couple already has boys and would like a girl, or vice versa, and so they go through IVF for the privilege of choosing the sex.

Not every clinic will do sex selection, and some clinics will do it only under limited circumstances, such as when a parent is a carrier of a disease known to affect only one sex or the other. Some will do it for "family balancing," when a couple already has boys and wants a girl or vice versa. The media has dubbed the result of this technology "designer babies." It is likely to go further in the future—eventually, you can know the color of your baby's eyes or hair before the embryo is implanted, but it's unlikely that you'll ever be able to pick more than one characteristic—not only is it asking a lot of science to identify each of these genes, but you also have to find embryos that contain just the right combination that the recipient wants—and you're not dealing with an infinite number of embryos. It's unlikely, for instance, for you to find an embryo that's male with brown eyes and blond hair when you have only six embryos to choose from.

# Premature Ovarian Failure

Premature ovarian failure (POF), also known as primary ovarian insufficiency, is defined as the loss of normal ovarian function before a woman turns forty. It's a rare condition affecting about 1 percent of women of reproductive age. There's still a 1–2 percent chance that a woman with this condition will get pregnant without interventions—there is still irregular ovulation and menstruation, which leaves the slim possibility open. It's not quite the same thing as premature menopause, which is when all ovarian function has stopped and pregnancy is no longer possible. But still, the odds are very low and we haven't come up with any way to fix it. Until now.

In vitro activation (IVA) is a new procedure started in Japan, following successful animal studies. In this procedure, ovarian tissue is first removed using laparoscopy and cut up into pieces. This disrupts the normal biological processes that would stop the tissue from growing. Then the pieces are treated with medication to "activate" the dormant follicles, and then grafted back into the woman. It requires two surgeries (to remove the ovarian tissue and then put it back), followed by IVF, so the costs are high and it carries the inherent risk of surgery. However, it also gives women with POF an increased possibility of pregnancy with their own eggs.

In the first experimental trial of twenty-seven women in Japan, doctors found that eight of the women responded to treatment: They had rapid follicle growth after the treatment. Of them, five women produced mature eggs, which were then retrieved. (Following this procedure, a patient's only option is egg retrieval and IVF.) The team's published report in 2013 indicates that one healthy baby has been born so far to one of their study participants. Another is pregnant as of this writing, one had an unsuccessful IVF cycle and two others have frozen embryos.

IVA doesn't fix the problem of age-related decline in quality and quantity of eggs. Thus far, it's been tried only to treat the problem of premature ovarian failure. And obviously, five egg retrievals and two pregnancies out of twenty-seven participants aren't huge numbers—but it's a start. It's possible that the technique needs to be honed, but that the principles are a great starting point and better odds than what the women would have likely achieved naturally.

We're not yet ready to try this treatment in the United States. So far, it's offered only in Japan, and it will probably be years before it's approved as a treatment in the United States (if at all), but it's an exciting new development that can provide hope for a population with an otherwise bleak fertility outlook.

# Uterus Transplants

For women with the congenital disease Mayer-Rokitansky-Küster-Hauser (MRKH) and for women who've needed to have their uteruses removed, there is a glimmer of hope on the horizon in the form of uterus transplants.

The first successful uterus transplant was performed on a woman in Turkey named Derya Sert in 2011. She was able to get pregnant following IVF, but miscarried after two months. The only other known uterus transplant before 2012 was in Saudi Arabia and the transplanted uterus had to be removed after three months due to blood clots.

However, a team of researchers in Sweden have just performed nine uterus transplants using live donors—family members of the recipients—and are hopeful that they will have the first baby delivered as a result of a transplant. They waited a year post-transplant before beginning IVF on each of the women, and the plan in each case is for the uterus to be removed after one or two successful pregnancies so that the recipient doesn't have to be on immunosuppressive drugs for the rest of her life.

There are significant risks inherent in this procedure, both to the recipient and the live donor, and numerous ethical questions involved. We also have no idea if a transplanted uterus can sustain a pregnancy—will the fetus be strong enough to grow for nine months and not get rejected, especially considering that not all of the blood vessels will be intact? Will the placenta be developed enough to nourish the baby? Will the antirejection drugs harm the baby?

Jamie and his team began studying uterus transplant years ago, beginning with rats. There have, in fact, been many animal studies that have shown that animals can successfully carry babies from transplanted uteruses. Once they got to human studies, though, they found that some issues were insurmountable—most notably, the immuno-suppressant drugs required for the transplant. There will always be people willing to take risks—doctors who want to be pioneers, and patients for whom carrying a baby of their own seems to outweigh everything else—but he decided that exposing a fetus to the medicines was not acceptable.

The speed of progress in fertility treatment is amazing, however, and there is still the chance that transplanted wombs will become a viable option in the future. These nine Swedish women may teach us quite a bit about how pregnancy works in a transplanted uterus.

The cool thing about this field is that it makes the impossible possible, and the technology is getting better all the time.

# Afterword:
## Toward a New Fertility Mind-Set

What it really comes down to is this: There are some things you can control about your fertility and some things you can't. You can do everything right and still not wind up getting or staying pregnant. And some women do it all wrong and seemingly have babies at the drop of a hat. It's not fair. It's not fair that drug addicts and prostitutes and abusive parents can have babies they don't even want. But life is not fair, and we can't let ourselves get caught up in that kind of thinking. What matters is that we do whatever we can do to get the best outcome and then adjust course as necessary.

There are thirty-seven different ways to make a baby now: artificial insemination, donor egg, donor sperm, surrogate, and so on. If you are determined to be a parent, then one of these ways will work for you. It may not be the way you always imagined, but taking a different path doesn't make you any less a parent and doesn't make your baby any less valid. Sure, there are some people who will judge you for your choices, but those people don't get a vote. We each get to carve out our own road in life.

We hope that you've learned a lot about the things you can do to preserve your fertility as long as possible, and that you will be happy and fulfilled wherever your path may take you.

# Resources

## Websites You Can Trust

The internet is a wonderful tool for fertility information—especially considering how quickly this field advances and how much there is to learn. However, it's also a giant cesspool of misinformation if you don't know where to look. Below are sites we trust that you may find helpful on your journey:

American Fertility Association: www.theafa.org

American Society for Reproductive Medicine: www.asrm.org

Centers for Disease Control and Prevention: www.cdc.gov

Endometriosis Foundation: www.endofound.org

Family Equality Council: www.familyequality.org

Fertile Thoughts: www.fertilethoughts.com

Fertility Authority: www.fertilityauthority.com

Fertility Planit: www.fertilityplanit.com

Fertility within Reach: www.fertilitywithinreach.org

Medical News Today: www.medicalnewstoday.com/categories/fertility

National Fertility Association: www.resolve.org

NYU Fertility Center: www.nyufertilitycenter.org

Our Bodies Ourselves: www.ourbodiesourselves.org

Society for Assisted Reproductive Technology: www.sart.org

Taking Charge of Your Fertility: www.tcoyf.com

# Keratin Brands to Avoid

This is not an all-inclusive list, but OSHA and a team of researchers have found formaldehyde at levels above 0.1 percent in each of the following products:

## Brazilian Blowout
- Acai Professional Smoothing Solution
- Professional Brazilian Blowout Solution

## Brazilian Gloss
- Keratin Smoothing Gloss

## Cadiveu
- Brasil Cacau
- Acai Therapy

## Chocolate
- Extreme De-Frizzing Treatment

## Copomon/Coppola
- Keratin Complex Smoothing Therapy
- Natural Keratin Smoothing Treatment
- Natural Keratin Smoothing Treatment Blonde
- Express Blow Out

## Global Keratin

## Gold Solution

# Kera Green Keratin

# Keratin Express

- Brazilian Smoother

# Marcia Teixeira

- Brazilian Keratin Treatment
- Advanced Brazilian Keratin Treatment
- Chocolate Extreme De-Frizzing Treatment
- Soft Gentle Smoothing Treatment
- Soft Chocolate Gentle Smoothing Treatment

# QOD

# Notes

## Chapter 1: Baby, Maybe

1. Centers for Disease Control and Prevention, National Survey of Family Growth (January 2014).

## Chapter 2: Sex and Fertility

1. A. Idahl et al., "Demonstration of Chlamydia Trachomatis IgG Antibodies in the Male Partner of the Infertile Couple Is Correlated with a Reduced Likelihood of Achieving Pregnancy," *Human Reproduction* 19, no. 5 (May 2004): 1121–1126.

2. Centers for Disease Control and Prevention, "Pelvic Inflammatory Disease (PID) Fact Sheet" (updated March 2014).

## Chapter 4: Lifestyle Differences for Fertility

1. American Society for Reproductive Medicine, "Patient's Fact Sheet: Smoking and Infertility" (2003).

2. L. Wise et al., "A Prospective Cohort Study of Physical Activity and Time to Pregnancy," *Fertility and Sterility* 97, no. 5 (May 2012): 1136–1142.

3. A. Scranton, "Chem Fatale," *Women's Voices for the Earth* special report (November 2013).

## Chapter 5: Medications and Health Conditions That Can Affect Your Fertility

1. G. Currier and G. Simpson, "Psychopharmacology: Antipsychotic Medications and Fertility," *Psychiatric Services* 49, no. 2 (1998): 175–176.

2. J. R. Bostwick, S. K. Guthrie and V. L. Ellingrod, "Antipsychotic-Induced Hyperprolactinemia," *Pharmacotherapy* 29, no. 1 (January 2009): 64–73.

3. S. C. Sukumaran, P. S. Sarma and S. V. Thomas, "Polytherapy Increases the Risk of Infertility in Women with Epilepsy," *Neurology* 75, no. 15 (October 2010): 1351–1355.

4. J. E. Chavarro et al., "Iron Intake and Risk of Ovulatory Infertility," *Obstetrics and Gynecology* 108, no. 5 (November 2006): 1145–1152.

5. American Society for Reproductive Medicine, "Fact Sheet: Endometriosis: Does It Cause Infertility?" (revised 2012).

6. R. Hart, "Gum Disease Can Increase the Time It Takes to Become Pregnant," European Society of Human Reproduction and Embryology presentation, Stockholm, Sweden (July 2011).

## Chapter 6: Don't Drink That, Put Down That Lipstick and Change Your Shower Curtain

1. A. S. Al-Hiyasat et al., "Effects of Bisphenol A on Adult Male Mouse Fertility," *European Journal of Oral Sciences* 110, no. 2 (April 2002): 163–167.

2. Y. M. Zheng et al., "Association between Serum Bisphenol-A and Recurrent Spontaneous Abortion: A 1:2 Case-Control Study, China," *Zhonghua Liu Xing Bing Xue Za Zhi* 33, no. 8 (August 2012): 841–845.

3. R. Lathi et al., Presentation at the annual meeting of the International Federation of Fertility Societies and the American Society for Reproductive Medicine, Boston, Massachusetts (October 2013).

4. H. Shu et al., "PVC-Flooring at Home and Development of Asthma among Young Children in Sweden: A 10-Year Follow-Up," *Indoor Air* (October 2013), epub ahead of print.

5. K. W. Smith et al., "Urinary Paraben Concentrations and Ovarian Aging among Women from a Fertility Center," *Environmental Health Perspectives* (August 2013), epub ahead of print.

6. A. Plenge-Bonig and W. Karmaus, "Exposure to Toluene in the Printing Industry Is Associated with Subfecundity in Women but Not in Men," *Occupational and Environmental Medicine* 56, no. 7 (July 1999): 443–448.

7. Wisconsin Department of Health Services, "Fact Sheet: Benzene" (revised 2012).

8. E. D. Pellizzari et al., "Purgeable Organic Compounds in Mother's Milk," *Bulletin of Environmental Contamination and Toxicology* 28, no. 3 (March 1982), 322–328.

9. Occupational Safety and Health Administration, "Fact Sheet: Hazard Alert Update: Hair Smoothing Products that Could Release Formaldehyde" (updated September 2011).

## Chapter 7: Eat, Drink and Be Fertile

1. C. Fei et al., "Maternal Levels of Perfluorinated Chemicals and Subfecundity," *Human Reproduction*, doi:10.1093/humrep/den490; first published online January 2009.

## Chapter 9: BMI and Fertility

1. J. Bellver, "Female Obesity Linked to Lower Rates of Live Birth and Embryo Implantation in the Uterus," first presented at European Society of Human Reproduction and Embryology annual meeting, London, UK (July 10, 2013).

2. P. Krakowiak et al., "Maternal Metabolic Conditions and Risk for Autism and Other Neurodevelopmental Disorders," *Pediatrics*, published online April 9, 2012.

## Chapter 10: Rumors, Myths and Truths about Fertility

1. J. Gaskins et al., "Physical Activity and Television Watching in Relation to Semen Quality in Young Men," *British Journal of Sports Medicine* (February 2013), epub ahead of print.

2. E. Levitas et al., "Seasonal Variations of Human Sperm Cells among 6455 Semen Samples: A Plausible Explanation of a Seasonal Birth Pattern," *American Journal of Obstetrics & Gynecology* 208, no. 5 (May 2013): 406. e1–406.e6.

3. R. R. Baker, "Copulation, Masturbation and Infidelity," *New Aspects of Human Ethology* (1997): 163-188.

## Chapter 11: When You're Ready to Start Trying

1. J. Boivin and L. Schmidt, "Infertility-Related Stress in Men and Women Predicts Treatment Outcome 1 Year Later," *Fertility and Sterility* 83, no. 6 (June 2005): 1745–1752.

2. H. Klonoff-Cohen, E. Chu, L. Natarjan and W. Sieber, "A Prospective Study of Stress among Women Undergoing in Vitro Fertilization or Gamete Intrafallopian Transfer," *Fertility and Sterility* 76 (2001): 675–687.

## Chapter 13: Guys and Infertility: Hey, It's Not Just about Us

1. A. Kong et al., "Rate of De Novo Mutations and the Importance of Father's Age to Disease Risk," *Nature* 488 (August 23, 2012): 471–475.

2. T. K. Jensen et al., "Association of Sleep Disturbances with Reduced Semen Quality: A Cross-Sectional Study among 953 Healthy Young Danish Men," *American Journal of Epidemiology* 177, no. 10 (May 2013): 1027–1037.

3. S.S. Young et al., "The Association of Folate, Zinc and Antioxidant Intake with Sperm Aneuploidy in Healthy Non-Smoking Men," *Human Reproduction* 23, no. 5 (May 2008): 1014–1022.

4. A. E. Al-Sanafi et al., "Effect of Royal Jelly on Male Infertility," *Thi-Qar Medical Journal* 1, no. 1 (2007): 1–12.

# Acknowledgments

## From Kyra...

This book would not have been possible without the birth of my twins, Sage and Kellan. You two are my inspiration, my heart and my reason for existing and writing this book!

I love you, Mom and Pop, for the nurturing and devotion you give the twins. You are the most dedicated grandparents on the face of this earth.

Thank you, Jamie Grifo, for the gift of babies and for the gift of your friendship. Yes, I love my husband, but you are the amazing man that got me pregnant! You are also my loyal partner in this exhilarating book adventure!

Huge hugs and love to our editor Becca Hunt, our literary agent Lynn Johnston and our remarkable writer Jenna Glatzer. You three believed in me, Jamie, and our book, and we are so grateful for all of you!!

## From Jamie...

Through my longstanding and treasured friendship with John Roberts, I met Kyra and the colorful odyssey that resulted in this book: Kyra as friend, infertility patient, mother-of-twins and now writing partner who shares the same vision I do in bringing hope and information to our readers.

My deepest thanks to team TWLFP: our literary agent Lynn Johnston, our steadfast writer Jenna Glatzer, Marybeth Raymond who helped keep the message on track, and our editor Becca Hunt who effortlessly brought together all the parts to produce and publish our book.

# Index

*Page numbers of illustrations appear in italics.*

# About the Authors

Kyra Phillips is an award-winning journalist for CNN, serving four tours in Iraq and currently working for the investigative and documentary units. Her coverage about racial tensions in Jena, Louisiana, following the appearance of nooses at the town's high school earned her a top documentary award from the Society of Professional Journalists. Previously, she anchored HLN's *Raising America with Kyra Phillips* and led the network's 2012 election coverage. You can download her podcast, "The Mom Squad Show" on iHeart Radio, iTunes. She is married to fellow journalist John Roberts. They are proud parents of beautiful twins. (Thanks to Jamie!)

Jamie Grifo, MD, PhD, is the Program Director of the New York University (NYU) Fertility Center, one of the most successful fertility clinics in the country. He is also Director of Reproductive Endocrinology, and Professor of Obstetrics and Gynecology. His research efforts led to the first baby born in the United States using the embryo biopsy technique to screen for and avoid a genetic disease. Co-Director of the NYU Egg Freezing Program, his team has created one of the largest and most successful egg freezing programs in the world. As an award-winning scientist, he has had over 155 publications in peer-reviewed journals. Dr. Grifo has appeared on the *Today* show, *GMA*, *Oprah*, and in countless media outlets, including the *New York Times*, *Newsweek* and the *Wall Street Journal*.